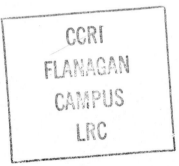

CONFRONTING DEATH

Medical Ethics series

David H. Smith and
Robert M. Veatch, Editors

CONFRONTING DEATH

RICHARD W. MOMEYER

INDIANA UNIVERSITY PRESS
Bloomington and Indianapolis

© 1988 by Richard W. Momeyer

Library of Congress Cataloging-in-Publication Data
Momeyer, Richard W., 1942–
Confronting death.
(Medical ethics series)
Bibliography: p.
Includes index.
1. Death. 2. Right to die. I. Title. II. Series.
BD444.M65 1988   179'.7   87-45439
ISBN 0-253-31403-8
1 2 3 4 5 92 91 90 89 88

To Alice Rhinesmith Schlundt
1944-1975

CONTENTS

ACKNOWLEDGMENTS

I have incurred many debts in writing this work, mostly as a result of the generosity of numerous persons, institutions, and organizations. The actual writing of the book began, peculiarly enough, with chapter one. This occurred in the winter and spring of 1981, when I enjoyed a research leave from Miami University and the hospitality of the Center for Bioethics of the Joseph and Rose Kennedy Institute of Ethics at Georgetown University. But I did not conceive of "Death Mystiques: Denial, Acceptance, Rebellion" as a chapter in a book until later in that year when I was fortunate to participate in a National Endowment for the Humanities yearlong seminar on bioethics, directed by David Smith at Indiana University. There, with the encouragement of a very able and critically supportive group of Fellows and Director, I first began to suppose there was sufficient continuity and coherence in what I was thinking to write a book. Chapters four and ten were drafted during that academic year of 1981–82; chapter three was sketched.

In the summer of 1982, a Faculty Development Award from the Woodrow Wilson National Fellowship Foundation allowed me to spend most days trailing about Will Leder, an oncologist in private practice, as he made rounds through Christ and Deaconess Hospitals in Cincinnati. This enabled me to extend and vary my observation of clinical practice begun more than a year earlier on the Oncology Service of Georgetown University Hospital. Still later, in May and June of 1985, I received an Exxon Foundation Fellowship in Clinical Medical Ethics to participate, with nine other teachers, in a series of seminars conducted by the faculty of the Center for Ethics, Medicine, and Public Issues of the Baylor College of Medicine. Along with these seminars went extensive observation and interrogation of physicians and nurses at work in the many hospitals of the Texas Medical Center in Houston. In all these settings, I wrote no more than notes, and learned an enormous amount: from sensitive, caring physicians and nurses; from stimulating teachers; and from generous, often dying, patients.

In the summer of 1983, I hid in my office and wrote chapters two and three and did preliminary research for chapters five and six. This work was supported by a Summer Research Award from the Miami University Faculty Research Committee.

A conference I organized for September 1984 at the Marcum Conference Center of Miami University, on "Treatment Refusal and Suicide: Medical, Moral and Legal Issues," had a profound effect on two of the chapters. First of all, Dax Cowart came as keynote speaker, and that caused me to think through much of what is said about his situation in chapter nine. Second, the conference ended with a panel discussion by David Jackson, David Smith, and Stuart Youngner that greatly stimulated my thinking on Joseph Saikewicz's case, discussed in chapter ten.

The largest part of the book—chapters five, six, seven, eight, and nine—was written in England, in the second half of 1986. A mostly research appointment for me as a Visiting Scholar to the Miami University European Center in Luxembourg, a leave of absence as Director of Butler County Planned Parenthood for Sue Momeyer, and absence with nominal approval from the Talawanda School System for Alison and Alexis, allowed us to make a home in London. There I spent most days in the Nuffield Library of the British Medical Association, where very knowledgeable and helpful librarians, and a magnificent setting, provided ideal conditions for thinking and writing. I did some of my work at the London School of Economics, where an affiliation as an Academic Visitor in the Department of Philosophy gave me ready access to computers for editing text.

A number of persons have read part or all of this work in manuscript and offered thoughtful, useful, and probably too often ignored suggestions for making changes. These include most especially Dax Cowart, Robert Burt, Sue Momeyer, David Smith, and Robert Veatch.

Among the deeper roots of this work is the experience I have had now for nearly twelve years at Miami University of teaching an interdisciplinary humanities course entitled "Confronting Death." This has been a consistently powerful and moving experience for me, and I have learned enormously from the colleagues I have been privileged to teach with and the students who have shared their experience and thinking. My co-teachers in this venture have been Roy Bowen Ward, religion; Roland Duerksen and Rebecca Lukens, English; Roger Knudson, psychology; and Terry Perlin, interdisciplinary studies. Among the students deserving of special mention are Chris Vinson, Ken McDiffet, and Kathy Boynton.

Earlier versions of chapters one, four, and ten appeared in the following publications, each of which has graciously granted republication permission: chapter one, in *Mosaic: A Journal for the Interdisciplinary Study of Literature*, February 1982; chapter four, in *Omega: The Journal of Death and Dying*, June 1985; chapter ten, in *Theoretical Medicine*, October 1983, and in *Bioethics Reporter*, September 1985.

The epigraph for chapter one, from the *Poems of Dylan Thomas*, copyright © 1952, is reproduced here by permission of New Directions Corporation. The final stanza of "Dirge Without Music" by Edna St. Vincent Millay, reprinted in chapter one by permission, is from *Collected Poems*, Harper & Row, copyright © 1928, 1955 by Edna St. Vincent Millay and Norma Millay Ellis. The epigraph for chapter three is from "Sweeney Agonistes," in *Collected Poems 1901–1962* by T. S. Eliot, copyright 1936 by Harcourt Brace Jovanovich, Inc., copyright © 1963, 1964 by T. S. Eliot, reprinted by permission of the publisher.

PREFACE

This is a book about the choices all of us must make in confronting death. Some few of these choices concern ourselves only; most directly and intimately involve others as well. Sometimes these choices are as fundamental as whether to go on with life at all; more often they have to do with our attitudes, feelings, and thoughts about life, its possible purposes and direction. Thus this is also a book about the values that inform the choices we make in life, during dying, and about death itself.

The reader is entitled to know the biases and commitments of an author on such matters as these. Most of mine, I hope, emerge clearly enough in the discussions on how people approach death and how they might best do so; on whether death should be regarded as a good thing, or immortality as desirable; on whether we ought to regard death as fearful or the fear of death as a worrisome inhibitor of giving good care to the dying, and so on. But it might still be useful to articulate at the outset some of my own most basic values that lead these discussions in the directions they take.

The questions taken up in this work are suffused with, immersed in, a long history of religious concern. No reflection on death, on meaning, on good and evil, on suicide and how to value life, on choices to resist death or submit to fate, can escape such a history. Nor would I want to ignore this dimension in discussing these topics. Nonetheless, I have done my best to shape and answer questions about such matters from a consistently secular point of view. This means that I have tried not to presuppose the need for or the truth of explicitly theological premises; further, that it has sometimes been desirable, even necessary, to assume the falsity of such claims; and finally, that on some occasions argument as to the falsity of theological premises is appropriate.

But while this is done unambiguously, it is not done without ambivalence. While I have little difficulty in rejecting fundamental religious claims—that there is a God, that individual human beings might survive the destruction of their bodies, that life without religious faith is meaningless, and the like—I do not dissent from some of the normative conclusions frequently thought to follow from such premises. That is, the religious traditions whose theologies I unambiguously reject have also used these fundamental beliefs to draw some normative conclusions and imply some values that I find far less problematical. Among these are an emphasis upon the value of each individual human life; the importance of caring for persons, especially impaired and vulnerable persons; and the need for drawing one's circle of moral concern considerably wider than one's own self-interest.

A reflective reader will have more difficulty discerning what I accept and advocate, as distinct from what I reject and argue against. This will not be your failure. The difficulty is largely mine. To put the matter rather crudely, if we can call the theological commitments sketched above a kind of "religious communitarianism," then its predominant alternative, in our culture and in our times, is a kind of "secular individualism." And it is the "individualism," rather than "secular," which I regard with the greatest ambivalence.

"Individualism" means many different things, but at the core of its central uses it denotes a moral commitment to regarding individual human lives as requiring respect, and individual liberty, often cast as "personal autonomy," as among the highest values. The first part of this coupling is for me the least troublesome: indeed, without the centrality of respect for individual life I do not think morality even possible. The second part is problematical, for it is not at all clear to me that respecting persons necessarily means valuing their freedom and self-determination above all other interests, either of theirs or of larger communities.

I thus find myself frequently attempting to tread a narrow path between two extremes: on the one hand is the ideology that values maintenance and nurturing of human life over all else, and frequently finds itself expressed in absolutist and religious terms as "the sanctity of life"; on the other hand is the ideology that supposes that only self-determination and individual liberty are adequate for defining the value of any particular life, and which itself is expressed in relativistic and libertarian terms. In attempting to thread my way between these views, I alternately tilt one direction or the other. Thus on the issue of whether death is always an evil for one who dies, I argue that it is. Nonetheless, I argue as well that it is one's right to make a wide range of choices for death, and that such a right cannot be legitimately restricted for any but the most compelling reasons.

Some draw from the view that human life is precious and of paramount value the implication that all forms of human life ought to be preserved as far as possible for as long as possible. This means that all choices for death—from abortion to suicide, from terminating life-prolonging treatment for those who wish such termination to surrogate decisions to end such treatment made on behalf of terminally ill persons incapable of making their wishes known—are morally indefensible. In the other camp, the most enthusiastic "individualists" are prone to suppose that life is valuable only so long as it is *valued*; hence, if the person whose life it is ceases, for whatever reason, to value life, there is little reason to think that person's choice to end life is morally problematical.

I share the view that human life is precious and of paramount importance, that each life has a value that may well exceed the valuing of it by oneself or by others. I think further, however, that human life is fraught with pain and suffering, that while human aspirations are virtually unlimited, our capacities for fulfillment are severely restricted, and that, all things considered, human life is pervasively tragic. Consequently, I do not believe there is any moral imperative to prolong all human life to the maximum degree possible. Other values—including, but not limited to, rights of self-determination—have a role to play in when death should be chosen. Frequently enough, there is not merely moral permissibility for hastening the end of life; doing so may well be obligatory.

In endorsing a broad range of morally legitimate choices for death, I am at pains to distance myself from those who take a rather benign view of dying and death, those who, in chapter one, I accuse of "romanticizing death." I find nothing appealing about death. There may be something good to be said for some sorts of dying—not much, but something, and then only *relative* to other ways of dying; there is still less to recommend death. The best that can be said for death, I argue, is that on some occasions certain forms of life would be worse than being dead. This still makes death an evil—in the requisite sense that for the one who dies the loss of life of any sort is a substantial, significant loss.

Another belief I hold, but do not much support in what follows, is that much of what justifies specially valuing human life—a view often thought to be blatantly "speciest"—is that in all of known nature human beings are unique. More than any other creature, human beings are self-defined, and to the degree that they are self-defined, they are also self-creating. Less than any other creature, we are determined by our biological natures. These unique capacities of human beings, expressed in the whole history of humankind through the creation of society, civilization, culture, knowledge, art, music, science, philosophy, *ad gloriam*, warrant placing especially high value on human life. Neither rationality nor consciousness alone suffices to make human life unique, but the achievements of rationality and consciousness make human beings something to be especially prized.

I think one way human beings are self-creating is in our tendency to push against that which limits our aspirations for creative achievement. Nothing more surely or universally restricts our transcendence of limits than death itself. Thus, insofar as self-creation and the attainment of our collective struggle for progress are good things, death is a bad thing. Further, resistance to death has much to recommend it, and so I find considerable merit in that approach to death called "rebellion."

Readers not sharing my perspectives will, I hope, still find merit in this work. One way in which this might be done is in working one's way through the analyses and arguments supporting the positions taken and those criticized. For outside these introductory remarks, I have struggled to support my views with argument, to take more the route of reasoned argument than profession of faith. I stop short of claiming Truth supported by Universal Reason for my positions, since such could be claimed with neither good conscience nor a straight face. But I believe that most of what follows will be found at least interesting and frequently provocative by those who dissent.

A more profound value that I hope will be achieved in this work is that it make a contribution to each of our efforts to attain the Socratic ideal of living the examined life. Someone has said that "death, like the sun, cannot be looked at steadily." To this we might add the observation that no more than can earthly things be seen without the illumination of the sun can life be understood without reflection on death. It is not for naught that generations of philosophers did their thinking at desks on which a human skull sat.

"Confronting death" is something of a fraud. No confrontation of death is distinct from a confrontation with life, and no reflection on death can escape contemplation of what it is about life that we value, what it is that makes life worthwhile—when it is so—and what sorts of relations we choose to have with other persons. Hence, reflection on death is an inescapable component of our struggle to lead an examined life. If what follows makes a contribution to this effort on the part of readers, it will have been worthwhile.

A final note on reading the text might be useful. I have tried to construct the book in such a way that each chapter can stand alone, yet at the same time each successive chapter constitutes a building block in an extended argument. Thus it is possible to read chapters selectively and out of order—sometimes even not at all. But to grasp the full thrust of where the arguments in each chapter are leading, it is best to read them all in order.

For example, chapter three, "If Immortality Were Possible, Would It Be Good?" is characterized as a "thought experiment" on the desirability of endless life. It can be read alone and out of context, or it can be skipped by the less philosophically inclined, or it can be read as the exploration of an implication of the thesis in chapter two that to die is always to suffer a significant harm. The same might be said of chapter four, "Fearing Death and Caring for the Dying," except that here it is the more abstrusely inclined who might be tempted to pass on this exercise in applied philosophy. Only chapter eight is essentially unintelligible if not read after chapter seven.

However any individual may choose to read this work, it is advisable to begin with the Introduction and Overview to acquire a sense of what follows. And before plunging into the concerns of Part II, "Choosing Death," I recommend perusing the brief Introduction to Part II that marks the transition from Part I to Part II and summarizes the concerns of chapters seven through ten.

INTRODUCTION AND OVERVIEW

There are a limited number of categories into which human approaches to death might fit. If we begin with a focus on subjective responses to one's own death, as I do, then I think these categories are best labeled denial, acceptance, and rebellion. The burden of chapter one is to clarify and analyze these approaches, characterized as "death mystiques," and to assess each for adequacy in meeting human needs. Contrary to conventional wisdom, I find the acceptance of death the most problematical, although there is not a great deal to be said for death denial. Rebellion, correctly understood, seems to me the most subtle and complex of human responses to the prospect of subjective annihilation, and it is the one I recommend, inasmuch as any can be recommended.

In defending rebellion, I do not intend to leave the impression that such is always and only the appropriate response to death, one's own or another's. But I do believe it to be legitimate, even morally defensible, as an enduring and continuing response to a wide range of dying and deaths. Rebellion is not merely a stage through which "mature" persons pass on their way to a more desirable set of attitudes toward death. But then neither is denial always so. Nor, for that matter, is acceptance what we all must strive to attain in our inevitable confrontations with death.

Each of these is an altogether appropriate, mature, and, if you like, moral response to some deaths in some circumstances at some times. In saying this I am not endorsing an open-ended relativism. I argue, in chapter one and throughout, that some approaches to death are clearly preferable to others. Much, however, turns on the particulars of each individual case; much also depends on those deep and abiding value commitments we make. Among these values, I believe, is an emphasis upon the importance of sustaining autonomous human lives.

The claim that rebellion is generally the most appropriate response to real or impending death would be greatly buttressed if it could be shown that death is always a significant personal loss to a person—even to persons whose living is terribly burdensome, even to persons with greatly diminished autonomy. Thus in chapter two I argue that, for the person who dies, death is always a significant loss, if only of the possibility for further life, and is therefore in this sense an "evil."

Now it might be supposed that if, as I have argued, death is always an evil, then it follows that deathlessness (or some form of immortality) must always be a good. Chapter three is a thought experiment on precisely this latter proposition. Crucial to assessing whether immortality would be a good thing are two concerns: first, what sort of "immortality" is being considered; second, exactly which and how many persons are we to suppose are immortal. My assessment of these questions leads to the conclusion that only endless, healthy, non-aging bodily existence is a plausible and potentially desirable form of immortality, but that with such immortality it makes all the difference whether a single individual survives death, or whether everyone does, or whether only some select elite continues. For an embodied immortal, it is not at all evident that any of these would provide circumstances in which endless life would be desirable.

Following this highly speculative thought experiment, I consider a much more practical implication of the argument that death is an evil. If to die is always to suffer a significant loss, then it seems to follow that to fear death would be altogether rational. This is an implication that I think is far more certain to follow than claims to the desirability of immortality. But some authors have contended that fearing death is an undesirable state, a less than rational response to annihilation, and a considerable disadvantage to those who bear any responsibility for caring for dying persons.

This last claim is one I examine at length. I argue that its force derives almost entirely from two errors. The first of these is a misconception about the nature and origins of human fears of death, the second a conceptual confusion that occurs when death anxiety is collapsed into the fear of death, and the fear of death is conflated with death denial. Once we get our meanings clear, however, the truth of the matter seems to me quite the reverse: unless one is acutely aware and sensitive to her or his own inescapable and rational fear of death, there is little prospect for being able to offer the best possible care to terminally ill persons.

If chapter three is a philosophical musing on logical possibilities and their desirability as far as the prospects for immortality are concerned, chapter four is an exercise in using philosophical analyses to clarify meaning and to offer direction on eminently practical matters. This is a duality that runs throughout the text: some discussions incline more to pure philosophical analyses—specifically, conceptual clarification—others are much more in the vein of applied philosophy, wherein clear understandings derived from such analyses are applied to problematical situations and argument is advanced to justify a specific action or attitude.

Chapters five and six incorporate both these tasks roughly equally. There is an enormous amount of conceptual muddle about such notions as "natural death" and "good death," and all the other phrases frequently used with them. Among these are such phrases as "death with dignity," "a right to die," "a right to die with dignity," and, to combine several of these already unclear notions into one perhaps irremediably confusing phrase, "a right to die a good and natural death with dignity." And yet for all the confusion engendered and questions begged by such language, there is much that is important and true that the use of these phrases, however ill-formed, is attempting to reach.

Thus I begin by considering what might be meant by asserting that

"A person has a right to a natural death with dignity." There are at least five distinct assertions contained here. The first of these is the claim that dying persons have a right to die with dignity rather than being treated as objects (diseases). Further, one who asserts "a right to die with dignity" may be advancing an ideal that everyone should aspire to, viz., that each of us should strive to maintain a sense of our own self-worth even as life wanes within us. Third, it might be that one intends to offer a guide to medical practice: "artificial means" of prolonging the lives of terminally ill patients are to be avoided. Fourth, to claim that a person has "a right to a natural death with dignity" may be to suggest that as a matter of public policy, legislation should be enacted to empower dying persons to exercise greater control over the circumstances of their death—for example, through funding hospices or legitimating "living wills." Finally, one who asserts "a right to a natural death with dignity" may be covertly advancing an argument for the "naturalness" of death and the desirability of each person coming to "accept" death for herself or himself.

In all five variations of the assertion that there is "a right to a natural death with dignity," the meaning of "natural" is central. I argue that when "natural" is carefully analyzed, one will discover enormous ambiguity in the term. In fact, there are six distinctly different relevant meanings of "natural" that must be sorted out: scientific, statistical, anthropological, conventional, theological, and evaluative.

After these have been sorted out, it is then possible to examine the equation of "natural death" with "good death" (or "natural dying" with "good dying"). In the end, I argue that equating "good dying" with "natural dying" and "good death" with "natural death" engenders only confusion or begs the important questions. I recommend we dispense with such discourse altogether and get on with directly attempting to comprehend how dying can be good.

Chapter six does this. Three paradigms of good dying are investigated: sudden death, "appropriate" death, and death with dignity. For reasons I hope will be convincing, only death with dignity emerges as a worthy ideal of good dying. Why this is so turns on both insuperable difficulties alleged to attach to its competitors, and on an analysis of human dignity. This analysis uncovers some very fundamental human goods and values, including consciousness, rationality, self-determination, bodily integrity and self-esteem. To preserve these is to enhance human dignity, and to preserve these in the course of dying is to make possible death with dignity. Because such fundamental human goods are tied up with dignity, dying with dignity emerges as a most admirable ideal.

With such an analysis in hand, we are well positioned to assess whether the discourse of death with dignity is adequate to do all it has been called upon to do. That is, can this analysis of dignified dying be used to support the assertion of a right to die with dignity, to articulate an ideal of good dying, to guide medical practice, to shape public policy and legislation, and to advance an argument for accepting death? For the most part, I believe it will, and I attempt to show this with respect to three different phenomena: the claim that there is a right to die with dignity, the problem of dying with dignity while being cared for by the practitioners of modern medicine, and the belief that dying with dignity is an ideal all should strive to attain.

This much completes Part I of Confronting Death, for we have explored at some length a number of vital connections between death, good, and evil. The transition from Part I to Part II marks a number of changes. In the largest sense, it might be viewed as a transition from the private to the public, or from personal values and choices to public morality and policy. Part II, "Choosing Death," focuses on moral arguments in the public domain, on issues and cases that move well beyond the boundaries of private choices. Moreover, if Part I is viewed as making an extended case for resistance to death, for protesting its intrusion into vital human lives, then Part II is an exploration of when choosing death is a prudent, morally permissible, or even wise course.

Choosing to die is, when made for oneself by oneself, always in some sense suicide. (I do not use "suicide" pejoratively.) Choosing death for others has many names, ranging from murder to euthanasia to self-defense, and so on. I am more interested here in variations on choices for one's own death than I am in choices to bring about the deaths of others. Accordingly, chapters seven and eight concern suicide and the question of whether there is anything like a fundamental human right to bring about an end to one's own life. Chapter nine is an extended case study of the plight of a young man who has compelling reason to choose death but finds himself coerced into not doing so. Finally, chapter ten explores one narrow slice of the vast domain of choosing death for others, viz., those situations in which there is morally sufficient reason to do so for persons whose best interests may well reside in such a choice but who cannot themselves so choose due to irredeemable incapacity.

By the time we get to such issues as this, we will have moved very far into considerations of public policy and legal deliberations. Indeed, chapter ten investigates more than half a dozen cases that are widely known precisely because they went to courts of law for resolution, including those of Karen Ann Quinlan, Brother Joseph Fox, Joseph Saikewicz, Edna Marie Leach, Mary Hier, and others. Some of the criticisms of court decisions offered are harsh, but much is at stake in these (frequently inappropriate) legal deliberations, including both individual lives and large issues of public policy.

A more detailed account of the contents of Part II can be found in the "Introduction to Part II." I hope this introduction and overview makes clear the structure of the work, especially the logic of its development. Further, there is every author's hope that the reader's appetite for finding out whether the author's stated intentions will be successfully realized is sufficiently whetted to proceed with reading the book.

CONFRONTING DEATH

Part I
Death, Good, and Evil

I

DEATH MYSTIQUES
DENIAL, ACCEPTANCE, REBELLION

> Do not go gentle into that good night,
> Old age should burn and rave at close of
> day;
> Rage, rage against the dying of the light.
>
> Though wise men at their end know dark
> is right,
> Because their words had forked no
> lightning they
> Do not go gentle into that good night.
>
> Dylan Thomas

It is a matter of continuing controversy, in both psychological theory and philosophy, whether the fear of death is a basic fear, or derivative from other, more fundamental emotions or states of being. Psychological theorists have often tended to favor the latter view, positing such varied phenomena as "infantile conflict" and "intrapsychic structural tensions" as the primary categories from which death anxiety is derivable.[1] In contrast, existentialist philosophers in particular have generally inclined toward the view that death anxiety is the "ontological core" of every fear.[2] Whatever the disagreements between philosophers and psychologists on the status of death anxiety, there is somewhat greater agreement about how the human species deals with this anxiety: by elaborate attempts to deny the reality and ultimacy of death.

The denial of death occurs both at the level of societal and cultural constructs and in each individual psyche. Whole theories of civilization have been predicated upon the premise that collectively human beings strive to deny their mortality.[3] Complex social rituals concerned with the preparation and disposal of the dead bear eloquent witness to these views.[4] Cultural myths, such as the Gilgamesh epic or the story of Adam and Eve, which attempt to account for the introduction of death into human affairs as a matter of accident or willfulness, are also evidence of a perhaps universal tendency of humans collectively to deny the inevitability of death. And, up until quite recently, in America even to talk of death was considered to be obscene and taboo.[5]

These theories, however, are largely beyond the scope of the present inquiry. Rather, I should like to focus attention upon more individual and personal responses to death, emphasizing some of the general strategies for confronting death that can be used by individuals. For if death denial is perhaps the chief or even, in the final analysis, the only strategy, there are at least two other general approaches that can be employed by individuals: acceptance and rebellion. Each of these approaches to death can be sufficiently elaborated to warrant the use of the term "death mystique," thereby signifying a set of related considerations that constitute more than an attitude and less than a philosophy, but each approach raises serious questions about the values with which we act and the choices we make in confronting death.

Denial

According to Elisabeth Kübler-Ross, denial is virtually everyone's first response to the cataclysmic news that they suffer a terminal illness.[6] This is as one would expect, for it is equally the response of one who receives stupendously good news. Something in each of us has trouble immediately accommodating a really shocking, surprising piece of information. But denial as a continuing response to the threat of death is another order of magnitude. It is that state of consciousness that finds it inconceivable genuinely to consider one's own demise: it is others who die, not I; I grieve for the loss of another, not at the reminder that I shall die.

Death denial at this level is less an action than an attitude or a psychological state, a way of coping with information that is disconcerting and threatening. It is a way of considering (or not considering) what we would rather not have to face, a strategy to protect ourselves from the loss of self-esteem, or of an important relationship, or of anything of value. At its extreme it requires extensive self-deception, a kind of lying to oneself that, paradoxically, involves simultaneously knowing something to be so and not believing it.[7]

The limitations of denial as a strategy for confronting death are self-evident. Trying to remain ignorant (not innocent) of the obvious is very difficult; rarely is it successful for long. Like other forms of lying, denial is hard to maintain consistently and constantly, and unless virtually everyone cooperates in maintaining the illusion, it fails.

Besides being difficult to maintain, denial ill prepares one for dying. Indeed, it might hasten death's arrival by occasioning the failure to take effective evasive action. Not being prepared for departure means a difficult exit, one that usually leaves much unfinished business behind. After death, of course, this is a matter of no concern to the deceased, but the dying itself can be unnecessarily strained by the failure to acknowledge what is happening. Denial, by inviting pretense and hypocrisy from all who attempt communication with the dying, taints precisely those relations it is intended to protect . And for the dying person, this social and personal falseness is one more painful burden, even if, ironically, he or she is responsible for the situation.

The third limitation of denial as a strategy for dealing with death is simply that it fails as a satisfying way of living. It violates that canon of wisdom conventionally attributed to Socrates: the unexamined life is not worth living. Precisely what death denial requires is that we not face and acknowledge the meaner realities of living, not just with respect to death and dying, but in all of our relationships and experiences. Denial and avoidance of unpleasantness—where dying is an ultimate unpleasantness—make for a superficial life, one perhaps conventionally respectable but finally hollow.

All of these themes are brilliantly illustrated by Tolstoy in "The Death of Ivan Ilych," beginning with Ivan's ability to accept the mortality of others but not his own. The syllogism he had learned from Kiezwetter's logic,

> 'Caius is a man; men are mortal; therefore Caius is mortal,' had always seemed to him correct as applied to Caius, but certainly not as applied to himself. That Caius—man in the abstract—was mortal was perfectly correct, but he was not Caius, not an abstract man, but a creature quite, quite separate from others.[8]

Similarly, denial of the fate facing Ivan is nearly ubiquitous. It is in every gesture, every motion, every social interaction; it permeates the atmosphere in the physician's office, in the law office, in the drawing room; between husband and wife, father and daughter, it is a heavy pall. Friends at the funeral fail to acknowledge to themselves what has happened; they are most inconvenienced by paying a call and missing a bridge game. Ivan's oldest boyhood acquaintance has a fleeting moment of recognition when Ivan's widow describes Ivan's final days of agony—and the great burden this was to her. But he soon rallies and returns to normal:

> "Three days of frightful suffering and then death! Why, that might suddenly, at any time, happen to me," he thought, and for a moment felt terrified. But—he did not himself know how—the customary reflection at once occurred to him that this had happened to Ivan Ilych and not to him, and that it should not and could not happen to him, and that to think that it could would be yielding to depression which he ought not to do. . . . After which reflection Peter Ivanovich felt reassured, and began to ask with interest about the details of Ivan Ilych's death, as though death was an accident natural to Ivan Ilych but certainly not to himself. (p. 102)

Ivan himself was able to keep the obvious from himself for a very long time, both because he devoutly desired to do so and because nearly everyone around him tacitly conspired in the deception that he was not dying. Only Gerasim, the simple peasant, the youthful, cheerful, candid butler's assistant, offers genuineness, compassion, and companionship. It is not much, but it is all Ivan Ilych has in his dying. All the rest is falsity:

> This deception tortured him—their not wishing to admit what they all knew and what he knew, but wanting to lie to him concerning his terrible condition, and wishing and forcing him to participate in that lie. Those lies—enacted over him on the eve of his death and destined to degrade this awful solemn act to the level of their visitings, their curtains, their sturgeon for dinner—were a terrible agony for Ivan Ilych. And strangely enough, many times when they were going through their antics over him he had been within a hairbreadth of calling out to them: "Stop lying! You know and I know that I am dying. Then at least stop lying about it!" But he had never had the spirit to do it. The awful, terrible act of his dying was, he could see, reduced by those about him to the level of a casual, unpleasant, and almost indecorous incident (as if someone entered a drawing room diffusing an unpleasant odor) and this was done by that very decorum which he had served all his life long. He saw that no one felt for him because no one even wished to grasp his position. Only Gerasim recognized it and pitied him. And so Ivan Ilych felt at ease only with him. (pp. 137–38)

At the outset of the story, Tolstoy offers this initially puzzling, seemingly contradictory judgment: "Ivan Ilych's life had been most simple and most ordinary and therefore most terrible." (p. 104). But well before the story is completed, we understand that "The Death of Ivan Ilych" is a devastating critique of conventionality, of social graces functioning to obscure the harsher side of life, of shallowness and hypocrisy in human relationships, and of the finally unfulfilling pursuit of comfort, propriety, and decorum at the expense of seriousness, candor, and compassion.

Acceptance

If denial is such a dismal failure as a strategy for facing death, it might seem that a desirable alternative is to reach the point where one makes his or her peace with this inevitability and comes to accept death with equanimity. And indeed through the ages it has seemed to many that this is an obvious goal to be striven for. It is often supposed that the noblest achievement for a person is to attain an abiding sense of calm before the terror of annihilation. Thus Socrates and Plato, Epictetus and Seneca, and countless other philosophers urge the acceptance of death. Christianity is explicitly predicated upon the conquest of death, holding that in the resurrection of Jesus God has presaged a re-creation of each of us, such that while departure from this life might be fearsome it does not mean total, permanent personal extinction. In this way, we either overcome our fear and accept death, or at least diminish its significance. Consequently, it becomes a kind of idolatry to fear death excessively, attributing greater significance to death than it has in God's scheme.[9]

Contemporary manifestations of this ideology surface in the recent "death awareness" movement: in the rise of a science of death (thanatology) and of death counseling as a profession; in the development of numerous organizations concerned with death education and research; in the burgeoning of death-and-dying courses in colleges and even in high schools; and last but not least in the tendency of literary journals to devote special issues to the topic. Furthermore, a significant part of the "death awareness" movement has recently gone far beyond advocacy of openness about death to espouse what must be regarded as a mystique of acceptance.

Consider, for example, the death counselor who has mastered Kübler-Ross's generally insightful analysis of the stages of dying that terminal patients typically pass through. It is a small step (implicitly supported by Kübler-Ross) to go from regarding this analysis as a descriptive and empirical account to taking it as a prescriptive and normative bit of advice. Thus the counselor may come to see his task as being not only that of easing victims through the unpleasantness of dying but also that of engendering a state of accepting death—as inevitable, as final, and as desirable. Rather than commit any of those old sins of hiding death's imminence and fostering death-denying illusions, we seek to help people openly, sensitively, and knowingly to recognize their impending death. The counselor's premise is that candor and demystification will naturally and properly lead to accepting death.

Or consider the physician who has taken seriously the humanistic concerns about the propriety of continuing life-sustaining (or death-delaying) treatments for the terminally ill. Such a person may well become convinced that this care costs too much in the hardest moral currency of all: human suffering. As a consequence, she may become convinced that the patient would be better off dead than having to endure increasingly agonizing and ineffective treatments that merely prolong dying. In one or more of a myriad of ways, she can use her skills and authority to relieve the patient's suffering and expedite his death. This she may do on her own initiative, without taking counsel with colleagues, client, or relatives, believing that she has been true to the better part of enlightened contemporary moral opinion which sees prolonged suffering with no prospect of cure as worse than death itself and which regards the acceptance of death as preferable to continued trauma.

Finally, consider the academic who teaches a death-and-dying course. Above all he strives for honesty, thoroughness, rigor, and theoretical soundness in the consideration of death-related topics. As a sensitive teacher he wants students to confront the stark reality of death. To this end he selects the best literature, the most beautiful poetry, the most powerful films; he prepares eloquent lectures, organizes provocative panels, requires extensive self-examination and journal-keeping by students. His premise is that "knowledge" will make death comprehensible and thereby subject to control and ultimately acceptable.

The mystique of death acceptance, in short, lies precisely in this tendency to present death as no longer the enemy: avoidance, denial, anger, guilt, rebellion, irony, bitterness—any human response other than the acceptance of death is the enemy. Death, we are told, is not so bad, not nearly as bad as being unable or unwilling to live with death.

Clearly there is much to object to in the above scenarios. In the first place, there is the direct and discernible harm done to the counselor's client who is eased into death, the physician's patient who is sped along the way without any informed consent given to such treatment, and the teacher's student whose superficial familiarity with death is replaced by a thicker intellectual armor shielding the person from any deeply disturbing encounter with death.

As for the more intrinsic features of the mystique of acceptance that are objectionable, these are harder to define, because, unlike death denial perhaps, acceptance has no single or simple psychological or philosophical origin. Indeed, the view that each of us ought to confront his own death with equanimity follows from a confusing variety of very distinct and often incompatible world views. It can be the conclusion drawn from Eastern mysticism as well as from Western Enlightenment rationalism. A full-scale investigation of the underpinnings of an ideology of death acceptance might require considering mind-body dualism from Plato through Descartes to the present; the putative (and actual) implication of regarding death simply as a "natural" event; the coherence and plausibility of views that individual consciousness merges into a great cosmic unity at death; doctrines of the soul, of individual immortality and resurrection, and so on.

At the same time, however, one can focus one's objections by pointing out that however they may be represented, these views only arguably embody genuine acceptance of death. Most are better regarded as but sophisticated forms of death denial. This is true of any view that does not regard death as final, as the complete cessation of consciousness and personhood. Where death is conceived as "sleep" or as a transitory stage en route to a different state of being, either bodily or nonbodily, either individual or collective, but in all cases some form of continuing existence, it cannot be said that this is a position that urges the acceptance of death in the full-fledged sense of death as the end of existence.

Not all forms of advocacy of death acceptance are predicated upon the supposition that death is not final. For some varieties of Epicureanism and Stoicism, for Enlightenment rationalism and for contemporary secular naturalism, no doctrine of dualism or divine salvation lurks behind the acceptance of death. Something more nearly approaching the acceptance of death as the complete and total annihilation of self and self-consciousness is urged.

The temptation is to say that only some version of materialism makes possible death acceptance in the fullest sense; all idealisms and dualisms that seem to urge death acceptance can be shown in the final analysis to substitute for acceptance an expectation or at least hope that consciousness will continue. I think that as a general tendency this is true, but, like most such sweeping generalizations, it is false when applied to certain specific cases. Hegel, for instance, urges that we accommodate ourselves to finitude by identifying our life strivings with the interests of an ongoing community that embodies and sustains our goals even after our personal demise. Hegel offers no illusions that individuals survive in any form other than the results of their life's work and aspirations being embodied in an ongoing community. Yet Hegel's philosophy is definitive of (one form of) philosophical idealism.[10]

Be this as it may, what should be said of contemporary forms of death acceptance? There seem to be three grounds on which the acceptance of death is usually founded these days. The first is traditional mind-body dualism outside of an explicitly theological context; the second, religion—specifically, Christianity; and the third, a contemporary secular naturalism. The first view is found in the latest work of Kübler-Ross, whose recent book *Death: The Final Stage of Growth* posits an afterlife of tranquility. It is also implicit in those efforts to demonstrate that dying is really just passage to another form of life, as in Raymond Moody's *Life After Life*.[11] But about these first and second bases for urging equanimity before death I have said all I wish here in asking whether these are genuinely death acceptance.

One assumption often underlying an ideology of death acceptance is that death is not the greatest evil that can befall one, even if we understand death to be complete annihilation of the self. Initially this supposition lacks plausibility, for death is the deprivation of that condition (life) that makes experience of all other goods possible. Moreover, the loss of life is the loss of a unique good, for unlike other losses we might suffer, no compensation is possible. Not only has there been the loss of some valued object, but the very subject suffering this loss is itself destroyed.

On reflection, however, we can conceive of states of existence worse than nonexistence—perhaps that condition of nonconsciousness that concludes a long, slow, extremely painful deterioration, or the incessant suffering of intractable pain certain to be followed by death. Some kinds of dying can be worse than death, and for those persons faced with them, death becomes a welcome release. At least in a very straightforward way death becomes the lesser evil and the preferred choice.

If some such view as this lies behind the secular naturalists' advocacy of accepting death, there is much to be said for it. For one thing, it can prove a welcome counter to that absolutist view that holds death to be an unremitting evil and one always to be struggled against. Such views as the latter have given great encouragement to an obsessive kind of medicine conceived as a constant struggle against death. Behind such an ideology medicine has frequently been deterred from its more achievable goals. Excessive medical aggressiveness, supported by sophisticated technological interventions, can do great harm and often succeeds only in placing persons in precisely those situations where continued existence is a greater evil than death. A view that death is not the worst we may suffer is a useful antidote to these practices.[12]

It is my contention, however, that at the core of the mystique of death acceptance is not resignation to those tragic conditions which render death the lesser evil that may befall one but rather a notion that death may be a positive good. This sentiment lurks within some discussions of "the right to die" and of death with dignity; it is implicit in the approval of some forms of euthanasia and discussions of rational suicide. There seems here to be an impatience with suffering—not just terminal suffering, but any suffering—and a notion that anything which stops suffering, including even death itself, is a good thing. Beyond this is some sense of a good death that is one's due. As astute and longtime a student of death as Robert Kastenbaum claims to have detected a movement in which "pleasurable dying and glorious death may be major 'consumer demands' in the future."[13] People who have all their lives rejected hedonism and pleasure-seeking as the highest human good now find in their dying that they are urged to cease resisting death and accept the inevitable. Others who have known neither justice nor joy are told that in dying they will find equity and peace.

In these last sentences is to be found the clue to what is most political and most troublesome about the mystique of death acceptance. In the final analysis it urges the adoption of an attitude, not simply toward death but toward life and the world itself, that many will find inappropriate and some will find to be morally objectionable. To its more egregious form of regarding death as a positive good, almost everyone (everyone not committed to some form of death denial) can find objection. But even in its more temperate form of simply regarding death as a lesser evil, or as a "natural" event that must be accepted, the mystique of death acceptance advocates an essentially passive and complacent view toward the status quo. In this it runs the risk of serving some very dubious political interests. Generals with wars to wage, politicians with criminals to execute, industrialists with profits to maximize, and even clergy peddling paths to salvation can all make use of a more benign attitude toward death. But many will find morally compelling reasons for rejecting the status quo, and hence by implication for rejecting an approach to life that urges benign complacence, peacefulness, nonresistance, resignation, and acceptance. These persons will, with Edna St. Vincent Millay, protest:

> Down, down, down into the darkness of
>   the grave
> Gently they go, the beautiful, the
>   tender, the kind;
> Quietly they go, the intelligent, the
>   witty, the brave.
> I know. But I do not approve. And I am
>   not resigned.[14]

Sometimes the idea that we ought to accept death is supported by the claim that death is a natural event in life, and it is a "natural" inference from this fact that death must be rendered acceptable. Death for each of us may be inevitable, inescapable, and universal. It may thus be, in one sense of the term, "natural." But does it follow from this natural fact that I shall die that I ought to make my peace with death and be reconciled to extinction? What I have called "secular naturalism" draws this conclusion.[15] But I see no such necessary implication here. It is generally recognized today that it is neither a "natural fact" nor a "moral necessity" that there be only one kind of morally permissible sexual pleasure. Similarly, it is neither a natural fact nor a moral necessity that because death is inevitable the only reasonable response to it must be acceptance and equanimity. One of the things that may uniquely distinguish the human species is just our ability to choose how to respond to natural facts of sexuality and death. Nature herself (or God Himself) cannot reasonably be regarded as dictating the one right answer.

Rebellion

These reservations about the criticisms of accepting death lead to a final possible approach to death, and that is resistance or rebellion. Not resistance that constitutes death denial, and not rebellion that consists in vainly screaming at the skies, cursing the arbitrariness and "injustice" of the cosmos, but resistance rooted in the conviction that the world is not an altogether agreeable place for human beings (even despite there being no other); that not merely the collectively determined organization of human affairs is fraught with inequity and oppression, but the very structure of the "natural" order, in its ultimate indifference to humankind, is a cold and foreboding if not outright hostile place. The sensibility that underlies this mystique finds perhaps its angriest and most affirmative formulation in the closing lines of Simone de Beauvoir's account of the very difficult dying of her mother:

> There is no such thing as a natural death: nothing that happens to a man
> is ever natural, since his presence calls the world into question. All men
> must die: but for every man his death is an accident and, even if he knows
> it and consents to it, an unjustifiable violation.[16]

Rebellion against death, and against everything death symbolizes, is not a uniquely twentieth-century phenomenon, but it is one most pronounced and poignant in our time. No doubt this has much to do with the Promethean nightmare having become political reality: now it is possible, and many suppose increasingly likely, that humankind will succeed in the final destruction of the world. Beyond individual death anxiety, we have now also to contend with the increasing likelihood of total global extinction. Even the slim Hegelian hope of our individual strivings contributing to an ongoing social enterprise is threatened by the prospect of nuclear war. And in the light of these dangers only the foolhardy would urge complacence; for the rest of us, some serious commitment to prevent the realization of nuclear war is the only reasonable alternative.

As a model of anything but hysterical, panicked rebellion, we might look to the quiet, dogged, but unceasing resistance to death epitomized by some of the characters in Albert Camus's novel *The Plague*. Plague can be taken as an extended metaphor for any evil that threatens to overwhelm us, from Nazism to war to genocide to death itself. And the approach to these evils recommended by Camus—not just in the personage of the central character and narrator, Dr. Bernard Rieux, but also in that of his best friend Tarrou, and the ordinary clerk Joseph Grand—is far from dramatic or conventionally heroic.

Joseph Grand aspires above all else to write a novel that upon being read by a publisher will provoke the publisher to stand up and cry out: "Hats off, gentlemen!" But try as he will, Grand cannot get beyond the first sentence—cannot get it exactly right. And during the worst ravages of the plague in Oran, Grand's contribution is to keep meticulous mortality records. Yet it is Grand of whom Rieux (Camus) says: "if it is absolutely necessary that this narrative have a 'hero,' the narrator commends to his readers, with, to his thinking, perfect justice, this insignificant and absurd hero who had to his credit only a little goodness of heart and a seemingly absurd ideal."[17]

Tarrou, at first an enigmatic stranger, tells Rieux late in the novel and long after he has totally committed himself to the struggle against plague, "I had plague already, long before I came to this town and encountered it here. Which is tantamount to saying I'm like everybody else" (p. 222). Tarrou witnessed the execution of a convicted criminal by the state and was appalled. He spent years campaigning against capital punishment. But even so he concludes that his plague consisted of having had "an indirect hand in the deaths of thousands of people; that I'd even brought about their deaths by approving of acts and principles which could only end that way" (p. 227). Thereafter Tarrou resolves "to have no truck with anything which, directly or indirectly, for good reasons or for bad, brings death to anyone or justifies others putting him to death" (pp. 228–229). He vows always to take the side of the victim and, without believing in God, strives to learn how to be a saint.

For Tarrou, the only acceptable response to overwhelming evil, to undefeatable suffering and injustice, is to try not to do evil. This is not glorious or heroic. It is simply what is demanded of one who would be decent: never accept even unconquerable evil, but always struggle against it. Tarrou dies of plague nonetheless, and Rieux allows himself the following reflection:

> Tarrou had lost the match, as he put it. But what had he, Rieux, won? No more than the experience of having known plague and remembering it, of having known friendship and remembering it, of knowing affection and being destined one day to remember it. So all a man could win in the conflict between plague and life was knowledge and memories. But Tarrou, perhaps, would have called that winning the match. (p.262)

For Rieux himself, the struggle is constant and exhausting. The plague never dies or disappears; it is always with us. It cannot once and for all be defeated by some magnificent campaign; at best it may be held at bay a bit longer. Even though unwinnable, the battle must be joined: our individual integrity permits nothing less. What is required of us is not denial or resignation or acceptance, but a relentless human struggle, unaided by illusions of victory, against whatever form evil takes, including especially death. No doubt retreat will sometimes be appropriate (as when the mechanisms for continuing combat foster more plague than they cure), but surrender must never be declared. Camus concluded his novel with this penultimate remark:

> Dr. Rieux resolved to compile this chronicle, so that he should not be one of those who hold their peace but should bear witness in favor of those plague-stricken people; so that some memorial of the injustice and outrage done them might endure; and to state quite simply that there are more things to admire in men than to despise.
> Nonetheless, he knew that the tale he had to tell could not be one of a final victory. It could be only the record of what had to be done, and what assuredly would have to be done again in the never ending fight against terror and its relentless onslaughts, despite their personal afflictions, by all who, while unable to be saints but refusing to bow down to pestilences, strive their utmost to be healers. (p. 278)

Like the death mystiques of denial and acceptance, however, there are problems with rebellion. One of these is evident in the abundance of militaristic metaphors which characterize this approach. It is difficult to think in such language without creating illusions that our struggle will result in some sort of abiding victory. And yet this is exactly what we must do, for the point of the struggle is not to conquer death, but to assert our humanity, preserve our integrity, and affirm our dignity even in the face of the absurd assault upon them that death presents. Human dignity at its best is exemplified in the struggle against all that limits and oppresses men and women. This tension, and maintaining this tension, is at once the strength and the difficulty in the mystique of rebellion against death. While avoiding the romantic illusion of a Don Quixote, we are urged nonetheless to keep tilting at the windmills. Death rebellion requires keeping a delicate balance.

It would not be difficult to transform anger into resistance and resistance into a form of death denial. If we even suppose that our struggle against death might somehow succeed (or even should succeed in some enduring way), we slip into still another form of death denial. This is why I remarked at the outset that in the end it might be concluded that as far as human beings are concerned there are only variations on the theme of death denial. But while there is this danger that all human responses to death are ultimately variations on denial, there is no necessity that the danger be realized. For by now I hope it is clear that there are significant choices presented to each of us as to what kind of approach we will individually take to death. And the approach we take to death, not as a matter of psychological necessity or social conditioning but as a function of reflection and the search for self-knowledge, reveals our true selves as clearly as anything can. Nothing focuses the mind as death does. In choosing how to confront death, we choose how to confront life itself. And in that choice lies the very possibility of constructing one's own character and moral self.

II

IS DEATH AN EVIL?

> So death, the most terrifying of ills, is
> nothing to us, since so long as we exist,
> death is not with us; but when death
> comes, then we do not exist. It does not
> then concern either the living or the dead,
> since for the former it is not, and the latter
> are no more.
>
> Epicurus
> *Letter to Menoecus*

Perhaps no one today can fail to be struck by the oddness of the question that occasions this reflection. Throughout history the nearly unanimous response has been that death is surely an evil–if not always the greatest evil, then among the greatest, and assiduously to be avoided. In our unreflective moments we have no doubt that our own death is a great personal misfortune and is to be avoided at least as long as life retains its value for us. Moreover, we have collectively devised elaborate cultural and religious mythologies in attempts somehow to rationalize death, to explain how we come to be afflicted with the dreadful prospect of personal annihilation. Thus at the core of the dominant religion of Western culture are the teaching that death is God's punishment for humankind's sinfulness and the hope that redemption and eternal life are possible through divine grace.

But traditional accounts of the evil of death have lost much of their appeal and force in our time, and the question must be posed anew as to how to account for our compelling feeling that for each of us death is a terrible inevitability. An additional urgency in addressing this question is provided by the contemporary movement to romanticize death. Rooted in the phenomenon whereby some people live "too long" and die "too slowly" due to the use of a medical technology that usually serves us very well, the movement to romanticize death sometimes finds expression in such phrases as "death with dignity," "a right to die," and "natural death."

Furthermore, efforts to explicate a notion of natural death and draw from this "the counsels of finitude" pose the most sophisticated intellectual challenge to the notion of death as evil. For in such accounts as these, we are to suppose that the fact that each of us is born and will die provides a frame within which whatever story our lives tell must be completed. And precisely because our story is circumscribed by this finite frame, events in life take on at least a possibility of meaning that they would not otherwise possess.[1] In the face of all this, the times seem right for wholly secular and unromanticized efforts to shore up our preanalytic conviction that death is an evil. I intend this reflection as a modest contribution to that end.

Some points of preliminary clarification are necessary before progress is possible in considering whether death is an evil. First, and most easily done, is to assert that by death I really do mean death: the complete and total and final annihilation of an individual's personhood. No notion of transformation to another "state of being" lurks behind the bare-boned conception of death. With death comes the cessation of consciousness, not temporarily, but irreversibly; not even for some several millennia, but eternally. Whether immediately or with relative rapidity, with death comes also the deterioration and eventual destruction of one's body. Death is final; there is no surviving death.

Somewhat more problematical are the issues of what sense of 'evil' is intended, and for whom death is to be regarded as an evil. For both these I intend a very egocentric—albeit a rationally egocentric—point of view. By "evil" I mean "personal misfortune," so that to say of someone that they have suffered an evil is to say that something of great value to that person has been lost, or that an injury has been done to him or her. One may, of course, suffer such harms, injuries, and losses without being aware of it, without even minding it, although ordinarily it is our awareness and dislike of an event that helps make it an evil.

But suffering an evil in this sense is not simply a subjective matter of preferences or personal evaluations. What is at issue as well is whether there are objectively good reasons, available to all rational agents, for supposing death is a personal misfortune to the one who dies. So in asking whether death is an evil for an individual, I will not be asking merely whether any given person so regards death; I will in part at least be asking whether, from the perspective of an objective rationality, each of us ought to suppose that in some intelligible sense our own death is a personal misfortune, whether there is objectively good reason for rational persons to regard their own death as evil, however little, in our unique circumstances, each of us may feel it to be so.

It is worth remarking that this perspective, and even the conception of rationality with which we will be working, are very circumscribed. In any broader inquiry into death and evil, we would in all likelihood be led to quite different conclusions. For example, if we were to ask if the death of an individual person could reasonably be regarded as a harm or loss to specific other persons, our answer would require knowing a good deal about the relationships that obtained between the deceased and the survivors. And then if, still more generally, we were to ask whether a particular person's death were a loss to society, much would turn on who that individual was and what that person's contributions had been and might yet be expected to be. And if finally we were to ask our questions with respect to the interests of humanity considered as a natural biological kind, we would have to conclude that at worst the death of an individual was a matter of indifference, and that, for the most part, individual deaths are necessary to the maintenance of evolutionary processes in natural kinds and, in that respect, are a good thing. We have thus something of a continuum here in which as we move from subjective, egocentric individual evaluations of the status of death to more general and abstract perspectives our evaluation changes, perhaps even totally. For, as I will argue, it is always reasonable to regard a person's death as an evil suffered by that person, even though this death may or may not be an evil for others and is surely not so from the perspective of the interests of the species as a natural, evolving kind.

Death as Not Evil

There have been traditionally two often asserted arguments to show that death is not properly regarded as an evil for the person who dies. The first of these arguments was advanced at least as early as Plato's *Apology*, and is most familiar in the nearly aphoristic formulation given by Epicurus in his *Letter to Menoecus*.[2]

> So death, the most terrifying of ills, is nothing to us, since so long as we exist, death is not with us; but when death comes, then we do not exist. It does not then concern either the living or the dead, since for the former it is not, and the latter are no more.

Here we must suppose Epicurus to be advancing a serious argument for not fearing death rather than simply assuring his followers that they need not fear an afterlife. And we must assume that his characterization of death as "the most terrifying of ills" is a bit of ironic hyperbole. Both assumptions are historically problematical, but never mind. The sort of thing Epicurus says here can be advanced as a serious argument for not regarding one's own death as evil or properly fearful. So regarded, the argument runs as follows: Only that which is experienced as painful or otherwise undesirable is evil and fearful. But death is a condition in which nothing is experienced, for the subject of experience no longer exists. Hence, it is unreasonable to fear death.

In this argument, one should not be misled by the characterization of death as a "condition," for death is not a state of being, not even a state: it is nonexistence, annihilation of consciousness, the end of an experiencing subject. It is not "being in a condition" of death that one could even sensibly fear, but rather not being at all. But such a fear, this argument holds, is unreasonable, for there is no being left to experience deprivation.

A second argument to the same end holds that a longer or shorter than "normal" life-span is undesirable for humans, undesirable to the point of being an evil. Hence, it is not death that one ought reasonably to fear, but only death that comes too early or too late. Clearly this argument is less ambitious than the first, for it allows for the reasonableness of regarding death as an evil when it comes too soon. But it seeks to negate this evil once life has passed its "desirable" (natural, good) limit, and even to turn it around with the suggestion that beyond a certain point it is continued life that should most reasonably be regarded as a misfortune.[3]

Let us take the second argument and its essential claim first. On what grounds could it be maintained that too much life is undesirable? One ground might be that as life goes on its quality diminishes necessarily as a function of bodily aging and at least eventual mental deterioration. But this fact does not provide adequate support for the strong claim that death is not an evil and not to be feared, for that claim diminishes the supposed evil of death by shifting attention to the evils of aging. And it is open to one who disdains death to disdain deterioration as well and to maintain that such deterioration leading to death is but part of the same tragic reality that afflicts each of us. Death need not be thought less unfortunate just because it is preceded by other evils; it would be better still if neither deterioration nor death afflicted us and we could live on with health and vitality.

A better ground for supposing death at the proper time to be neither evil nor fearful is the claim that beyond a certain point life simply and inevitably becomes tedious, repetitious, and boring. Bernard Williams has advanced the most extensive and careful argument for this position, holding as he does that

> an endless life would be a meaningless one; and that we would have no reason for living eternally a human life. There is no desirable or significant property which life would have more of, or have more unqualifiedly, if we lasted forever.[4]

William's full argument for this position turns on the notion of "categorical desire," to be examined presently; at its core is the conviction that human satisfactions eventually give out: after a while experiences become repetitive and tedious and invariably boring. An endless array of such repetition would be worse than death; from such tedium death would be a welcome release. Williams seeks to show that such a development is not merely a contingent fact of human existence, it is inescapable.

Three responses to this view come to mind. The first is that there is a profound implausibility to it. The world is vast, variegated, and mysterious; there is no end to pursuing understanding, no lack of novelty, no stagnation in the world. If people ceased to age and die, much else would continue to change, not least the changes wrought by people, and there is no obvious reason to suppose such a dynamic process would necessitate tedious repetition and unbearable boredom. Secondly, mere repetition, even repetition of essentially identical experiences, does not necessarily lead to boredom. Consider satisfaction of the basic biological drives: so long as appetite remains strong, food and sexual union remain satisfying. It is in the very nature of such desires that they are self-renewing, never once and for all satiated and abandoned.

This leads to a third observation. It seems that Williams has covertly smuggled back into his reflections on human immortality the notion of aging, of decline, of deterioration. He wants to speculate on what endless life and lack of growing older would be like, but in the supposition that all repetition is tedious and ultimately boring he must suppose that such fundamental biological drives as those for food and sex decline or change, or how else could the process of satisfying them become boring? But if we suppose a lack of decline in intellectual vitality, in curiosity and wonder, and in more basic biological impulses, and couple these with the recognition that the world itself provides ceaseless opportunities for novelty and satisfaction, there would seem to be little reason to think endless life undesirable.

Consider now the first argument against the notion that one's own death is an evil, the argument I called "Epicurean." The counter to the Epicurean argument for not fearing death is itself the best reason for thinking death an evil. In his article "Death" Thomas Nagel seeks to show precisely how death is an evil. His thesis is that

> . . . it is good simply to be alive, even if one is undergoing terrible experiences. The situation is roughly this: There are elements which, if added to one's experience, make life better; there are other elements which, if added to one's experience, make life worse. But what remains when these are set aside is not merely neutral: it is emphatically positive. Therefore life is worth living even when the bad elements of experience are plentiful, and the good ones too meager to outweigh the bad ones on their own. The additional positive weight is supplied by experience itself, rather than by any of its contents.[5]

Nagel's view is that death is not an evil for any features it has, it is an evil because life is a good and death is the deprivation of that good. But this view encounters serious difficulties. One of these difficulties requires a direct response to Epicurus's assumption that nothing can be an evil to one who no longer exists. Another difficulty derives from applying the principle that no mere absence of a possible good can be an evil if there is no one who minds the deprivation.

Nagel first observes that there is a plentitude of evils that might befall a person even though that person remains ignorant of them—for example, deception, betrayal, being ridiculed behind one's back, and the like.

The crucial mistake in the supposition that one must mind an evil for it to be an evil is a confusion about time and relational properties; it is the assumption that "all goods and evils must be temporally assignable states of the person." But the truth of the matter is that

> most good and ill fortune has as its subject a person identified by his
> [sic, passim] history and his possibilities, rather than merely by his categor-
> ical state of the moment—and that while this subject can be exactly lo-
> cated in a sequence of places and times, the same is not necessarily true
> of the goods and ills that befall him. (p. 5)

If Nagel is right about this, it solves not only the difficulty about how one may suffer an unminded evil, but also the problem of how one who no longer exists can be said to have suffered the evil of death. For if at least some of the goods and evils that belong to a person are intelligibly separable from the actual condition of that person at a given moment, then we need not suppose that that person's being aware of these, or even that that person's continued existence, is necessary to speak sensibly of these as goods or evils for the person.

Nagel's illustration of these claims is apt. He asks us to imagine a man who has suffered brain damage to the point where he is reduced to the state of being a contented infant. Now only a dry diaper and a full stomach are required to sustain those pleasures of which he is capable. Has he suffered a misfortune? Most assuredly he has, despite not being able to mind his misfortune and despite the difficulties involved even in regarding this person as the same person whom we earlier knew as an intelligent, mature adult. The evil he has suffered is a loss of possibilities, of capacities and opportunities he would have had had he not suffered such grievous brain damage.

Death is an evil for one because it is the irrevocable loss of opportunity, of possibility, of the continued good of life. Death is a deprivation of life; were one not dead, one would be alive, and his or her possibilities for satisfying experiences could be realized.

One correction to Nagel's view is in order here. His argument so strongly shows death to be an evil that one is likely to be led to the view that it is the greatest evil one may suffer. And while this is often, even ordinarily, the case, it is not universally or necessarily true. Misfortunes of appalling variety plague human beings while they live, and sometimes the severity of these ills empties life of significance, of value, of the very possibility of regarding continued life as a good. This has implications for how we ought to regard some suicides, infanticides, senicides, etc. But it also, and here more relevantly, has implications for how we weigh the evil of death. For from some of the more severe misfortunes humankind may suffer, death is genuinely an escape and a release. The worst evils some suffer in this world precede death, and death, when it comes, may even be welcome. It might be said of Karen Ann Quinlan, for instance, that the worst thing in her life was not her death in June

1985, but that catastrophic injury a decade earlier which permanently emptied her life of vitality and consciousness and rendered her irretrievably comatose. And so it is, as well, with the elderly dying in our technologically sophisticated hospitals today: death may not be so great a personal misfortune as the loss of control, of awareness, of the capacity for communication, *ad nauseam*, that precedes death with intubation, tranquilization, artificial respiration and supported circulation, etc.

Having said all this, however, one must also note that the argument falls short of showing that death is ever not an evil. That it may not be the greatest evil some suffer makes it no less an evil. There is no comfort in the recognition that dying may be worse than death, that for some living may be worse than dying. It is not unreasonable for people to fear dying more than death. Many do. All this shows is that misfortune is inherent in the human condition. But that is no reason to think such a fate less tragic. And insofar as death is an evil of some degree at all times, it is always reasonable to regard death as an evil.

Life and Death, Good and Evil

Consider four logically possible, nonexhaustive, distinct valuations of death that might be proffered:

(A) Death is necessarily evil.
(B) Death is not necessarily evil, but is contingently so.
(C) Death is necessarily not evil; at worst it is neutral, a mere fact of human existence.
(D) Death is good.

Virtually no one holds D. To be sure, we do sometimes say of someone who has suffered greatly and experienced a prolonged dying that, for them, death is good. But what we mean by this is almost certainly nothing more than that in their case death is to be preferred to continued life of the sort found so objectionable, that death is a welcome release from a terrible dying. This view is entirely compatible with attitudes toward death displayed by both A and B.[6] Stoics have advanced C, and earlier I argued that this view is fraught with problems. Certain rationalists have as well inclined to C, for example, Spinoza, but their views frequently incorporate an emotional detachment to life that is unlikely to attract any who live without exclusively contemplating Truth, Beauty, and Goodness. The significant choice is between supposing death is necessarily evil, although not necessarily the greatest evil, and supposing that death is but a contingent evil, dependent, for example, on the balance of tolerable and intolerable, satisfying and unsatisfying, or pleasurable and painful experiences.

The choice between propositions A and B is a significant conceptual one that has received some attention in recent philosophical discussions of death.[7] One way to get to the status of death is to consider parallel propositions about the relation of life and good.

(A') Life is necessarily good.
(B') Life is not necessarily good, but is contingently so.
(C') Life is necessarily not good, but only a necessary condition of experiences which are either good or evil.
(D') Life is evil.

If we could say how it is that life is a good, we could know clearly what it means to say death is an evil. Here, as before, the significant choice is between the first two propositions: which of these better expresses an attitude toward life consistent with our deepest values? I shall argue that both A and A' are the more profound and adequate expressions of value, but in doing so I shall be at odds with some very astute defenses of B and B'.

The first, and crudest, position holds that life and good are contingently held together by a bond that exists for any given individual only so long as that person enjoys a net balance of good experiences over evil experiences. More or less sophisticated accounts might be given of what counts as good or bad experience (pleasure or pain, aesthetic sensibility or obtuseness, etc.), but the issue here is not the criteria for evaluating experience, but the simple calculation of which sort of experience is dominant.

Unfortunately, this way of attempting to link life and what makes life good does violence to our ordinary evaluations of when life is worthwhile. For in assessing the lives of others, we nearly always suppose that continued life, even with greater than ordinary suffering, deprivation, and hardship, is to be preferred to death. We typically regard the saving of such lives—whether in our own community or halfway around the globe—to be a benefit to the one saved. Moreover, we frequently regard those who opt for suicide in the face of temporary or even enduring misfortune as at least mistaken if for no other reason than that death is so permanent. No facile calculation of the balance of undesirable experience over good experience is likely to impress us into supposing that death is preferable to life.

Again, in assessing their own lives most people will continue to prefer continued life even in the face of the most severe hardship. Some cling desperately and many merely tenaciously; some fearfully and many more courageously; but nearly all people, when threatened and when suffering, cling to life. It may be that in some imaginable cases we are mistaken in doing so, and yet if we are, it is surely for reasons more profound than that at this point in our lives the balance of experience has tipped ever so slightly or even greatly toward suffering. So long as there is the slightest prospect of satisfying experience—not even a majority of such experience, but the possibility of it—human beings endure abysmal suffering and hope for more and better life. To turn around a popular cliché, it might be said that where there is hope, there is life. We admire, and we are right to admire, such power in the human spirit.

A far more sophisticated, but finally no more satisfying, position—that experience of any quality is a good to one having it—is Thomas Nagel's. As we have seen, Nagel holds that whatever other features it has, experience itself is always a good. There is no possibility of attempting to balance good experience against bad experience and arrive at a summary judgment, for all experience, *qua* human experience, is, as such, a good. Consider again Nagel's central claim:

> . . . it is good simply to be alive, even if one is undergoing terrible experiences . . . life is worth living even when the bad elements of experience are plentiful, and the good ones too meager to outweigh the bad ones on their own. The additional positive weight is supplied by experience itself, rather than by any of its contents. (p. 2)

But, as I alleged earlier, Nagel's view seems to go so far as to assert that life is an absolute good, which is a considerably stronger and less plausible claim than merely that life is necessarily good or, what amounts to the same thing, that life is intrinsically good. The difference between these claims is that if life were absolutely good, we would *prima facie* be justified in any effort, at whatever sacrifice and expense, without regard to all other (nonabsolute) values, to preserve an individual life. Even more strongly, we might be obligated to such ceaselessly heroic endeavors for the sake of sustaining any life, even at the cost of overwhelming suffering to the one whose life is sustained. Now few of us would go this far, though we would be willing to regard life as intrinsically good, meaning by that that life is desirable as an end in itself, that it has a value independent of the value of other things, including particular individual experiences or the balance of good and bad experience.

Moreover, it is an implication of Nagel's view that even a life of wholly negative experience would be a good. But, as Phillipa Foot asserts, this allows for a man's being slowly, agonizingly tortured to death being a good life.[8] Surely few people, under these circumstances, would doubt that for themselves an earlier, less painful death would be preferable to a longer life in which unremitting torture leads to certain death. There are thus circumstances of such singular horror that life under them cannot plausibly be regarded as a good.

Are we then back to supposing that it is merely a contingent fact that life is a good? Do we need merely a more plausible version of what those contingencies are that make life a good for oneself? A number of philosophers have supposed as much. Samuel Gorovitz, for instance, in an eloquent and insightful book, holds that

> It is reasonable to view one's own death as an evil so long as one is up
> to something one cares about with which it will interfere. Death may be
> no evil to the dead, but it can be an evil to the living. [9]

Gorovitz further denies that life itself has intrinsic value, because he believes an implication of this view is that it commits us to making every possible effort to sustain life, even the lives of the irrevocably comatose and in-
sentient. Life is a good only so long as some significant portion of life's
experiences are valued. As long as our lives are infused by meaningful
projects, we can speak of continued life as a good. But with the elimination of such vital activities passes as well the connection between life
and goodness.

Similarly, Bernard Williams thinks life good only so long as "categorical desire" endures. Categorical desires are those desires a person has
that are not conditional upon the assumption of his or her being alive. A
"rational, forward-looking calculation of suicide" would be a categorical
desire, for suicide is something one might desire which necessarily thereby excluded further life. As long as categorical desire exists, however,
death has a "disutility" for a person. But once categorical desire disappears (and in Williams's view, over a sufficiently long term it must necessarily disappear for human beings), it is continued life that is a misfortune. Hence, for both Gorovitz and Williams, the value of life is
dependent upon some feature ordinarily, but not necessarily, possessed
by experience. These features, called by Gorovitz "meaningful projects"
and by Williams "categorical desire," are what make life good, and their
absence—supposed somehow to be inevitable over a long enough time—
would empty life of significance and make death for one whose life has
been so impoverished no longer a loss.

Human Life as Intrinsically Good

It might be wondered, however, whether the connection between meaningful projects and categorical desire, on the one hand, and a life regarded as a good for one experiencing it, on the other, is all so accidental as Gorovitz and Williams suppose. (Williams, at least, has doubts
about this contingency, but does not develop them.) Could it not be the
case that unless human life possessed some such features as these we
would be mistaken in regarding it as human life, as the life of a person?
I suggest that those features of experience which make human lives
good are not merely contingently, but rather necessarily, connected to
our existence as persons. And I make this connection by arguing that
the notion of a fully human life is inherently a normative one, and that precisely what makes life human and personal are those features for which
there is consensus that they are essential to making life a good. [10]

In developing this argument, I suppose myself to be elaborating upon a suggestion of Phillipa Foot's, an elaboration for which of course Foot bears no responsibility. Foot writes that

> . . . there is a certain conceptual connection between life and good in the case of human beings . . . [I]t is not the mere state of being alive that can determine or itself count as a good, but rather life coming up to some standard of normality . . . Ordinary human lives, even very hard lives, contain a minimum of basic goods, but when these are absent the idea of life is no longer linked to that of good. [11]

Among those goods fundamental to a human standard of normality are the satisfaction of hunger, the opportunity for restful sleep, hopes for the future, work not demeaning or debilitating, and the support of family, friends, or community.

I think we need but take Foot's position one step further. Where she says that "Ordinary human lives . . . contain a minimum of basic goods, but when these are absent the idea of life is no longer linked to that of good," we could go on to say that when these minimum basic goods are absent, not only does the connection between life and good dissolve, but so too does that between life and human, or, put otherwise, so too does the connection between human life and the life of a person disappear. Without some such rock bottom minimum of that which makes life human and worthwhile, life is no longer human life. The same things which make life good make it distinctively the life of a person; their absence means not simply that life is no longer worthwhile, but that it is no longer human.

Human beings are uniquely distinguished from other creatures—if they are uniquely distinguished at all—by consciousness and its capacities and propensities to create projects, set goals, have an acute awareness of possibility and future, anticipate death, etc.—or in similar terms, by categorical desire and the ability to create meaningful projects. The absence of these capacities is not like the absence of other, less central goods, nor is the loss of other nonintellectual basic goods like the loss of lesser goods. Some losses destroy our very humanity. The connection of basic goods to human life is not simply accidental, but necessary. It is what makes life intrinsically good, and when life is thus intrinsically good, it is in the fullest sense *human* life. There is no fully human life, no life of a person, that is not intrinsically good. [12]

Vitalism and Dehumanization

Perhaps some light can be shed on these connections by considering two related concepts, those of vitalism and of dehumanization. Vitalism, in modern medicine at least, has come to be identified with "heroic" efforts to sustain life well beyond the point at which a particular life might

be of value even to the person whose life it is. Vitalism resolutely re-
fuses to make judgments or distinctions about the quality of life, preferring instead an adamant insistence on sustaining all life. Vitalists equate
human life with biological life: where there is the faintest semblance of
the latter, there is thought to be the former, and it is thought to be there
in such a fashion that every effort to sustain it is not merely permissible
but obligatory. In Rachels's terms, they see no distinction between being
alive and having a life. Hence vitalists typically allow no moral room for either abortion or expediting death.

As against this view, the one I have urged distinguishes "mere" biological life processes from that more complex notion of life that constitutes
the human. Yet this latter view has no automatic, immediate, or simple implications for when the termination of life is or is not permissible. This
is, at least in part, because the criteria for humanness are both vague
and slippery and always disputable in application. This leaves the door
open to a wide range of moral argument about when human life is present, and other arguments as to when life—fully human or otherwise—
may be terminated. But for nonvitalists holding something like the views
of humanness explicated here, it is clear that human life can be over
long before biological life ceases. This is the case with the irreversibly comatose ("brain dead"), whose vital biological processes may be sustained by drugs or machinery. It is more arguably the case as well with
the severely senile, with those who have suffered certain other kinds of extensive neurological impairment, with persons in ceaseless, uncontrollable, and unbearable pain, and so on with varying degrees of loss of humanness.

Dehumanization occurs when the deprivation of basic human goods is
extensive and profound. When the lives of human beings are reduced to
struggling to meet basic animal functions, for nourishment, rest, and little more, dehumanization is at its most intense. The model for how brutal and complete such dehumanization can be is the Nazi death camps.
Every possible atrocity, from terror to deprivation, from brutality to false
promises, was used systematically to deprive human beings of food,
rest, hope for the future, meaningful work, satisfying human relationships, and every other conceivable requirement for human life. Yet so in-
domitable was the will of some survivors that this very oppression fed a
will to live, to tell the story, to vindicate the victims. For this reason, the
fuller and more accurate conception of dehumanization applies to what
happens to oppressors, and not to the oppressed.

Dehumanization is two-edged: it affects victimizers as well as victims,
oppressors as much or more than the oppressed. To be the agent of attempts to denegate the dignity of others guarantees only one thing, and
that is not that one's intended victims will be made to live less than
human lives. What it far more certainly guarantees—as Socrates knew so
well and insisted upon so strongly—is that inflicting upon others such
harms as constitute dehumanization profoundly reduces the oppressor

to something less than human. Others may be demeaned and made to suffer indignity, but those who foster these ills are the more assuredly lacking in the moral sensibility and capacity for feeling vital to humanness.

If this account of what makes life an intrinsic good is a plausible one, it should suffice as well to establish the thesis of this chapter: that death is necessarily an evil for each of us. Death irrevocably deprives us of all possibility of more life, and since life, when it is human life, is good, the loss of that good is an evil. The loss of life, while always and necessarily an evil, is not at all always and necessarily the greatest evil human beings suffer. Some injuries are so utterly catastrophic, some suffering so intense, that while they may fall short of emptying life of its humanness, they nonetheless render death a welcome release.

Why Insist Death Is Necessarily Evil?

It might finally be wondered, however, that once this concession is made as to the relative evil of death, what is the point of still insisting that death and evil are necessarily, and not simply contingently, connected. I think there are several reasons for persisting in this claim. These reasons run from the abstractly philosophical to the practical.

One reason—an abstract philosophical one—is that this way of putting the matter gives us a deeper understanding of the concepts of life, death, goodness, and evil, and of the logical connections among all these notions. And that is no small matter, for among other things, wise action depends in significant part upon clear understanding. Understanding human life as necessarily or intrinsically good, as explicated here, and death as necessarily evil, allows for a deeper appreciation of the value that should be placed on human lives than other conceptions do. Perhaps this way of expressing the relations between life, death, evil, and good shows their connections better, and begs fewer questions, than do such notions as those of "categorical desire" (Williams), "meaningful projects" (Gorovitz), or a distinction between living and having a life (Rachels).

A second reason to insist that death and evil are necessarily connected has to do with a very subtle difference in moral perspective. If we suppose that life is but contingently good (and death but contingently evil), then the burden of proof for supposing any life good (or death evil) is upon the one who makes such a claim. This may not be a large burden or a difficult one in some cases; it is nonetheless a burden. On the other hand, supposing that life is intrinsically or necessarily good shifts the burden for establishing that conditions are such that in this particular case death is to be preferred to continued life. In modern medical contexts, for instance, judgments are frequently made as to whether it is desirable and worthwhile to use resources in the interest of sustaining a greatly impaired life. I think it far better that these choices be guided by the supposition that life is good and is to be sustained until proved otherwise. The analog in the law is that innocence is presumed until guilt is proven.

Now I do not think those who operate from the point of view I here characterize as less desirable are morally insensitive and eager to kill off other persons. We are not considering radically different moral points of view. Nonetheless, it seems to me that assuming anyone's death to be an evil until it is persuasively demonstrated to be at most a lesser evil affords a significantly greater degree of protection to the vulnerable, the weak, the powerless, in short, to all those not fully able to participate in making these judgments in their own cases. And the unhappy fact is that judgments about life's quality in situations in which choosing death is an option are almost always made by those whose own lives are not at stake. Hence, whatever small advantage can be provided the otherwise disadvantaged is to be morally preferred.

IF IMMORTALITY WERE POSSIBLE, WOULD IT BE GOOD?

> Birth, and copulation, and death.
> That's all the facts when you come to brass tacks:
> Birth, and copulation, and death.
>
> T.S. Eliot
> *Sweeney Agonistes*

The conclusion of the last chapter has some disturbing implications. If death is always an evil, even if not the worst evil one may suffer, it might be supposed that each of us would be better off if we *never* died. Thus immortality of some sort would be a desirable and rational goal. And yet very little reflection will show such an aspiration to be fraught with difficulties—so much so, in fact, that it may well seem that not dying would be as bad as dying. There is a paradox in the dual suppositions that death is an evil and deathlessness is too. We will need to explore this paradox, beginning with a thought experiment about immortality.

One of the most enduring hopes embodied in some of humankind's most pervasive myths has been that death be vanquished. Individually and collectively, we have hoped and dared to believe that death is an accident, a contingent fact for human beings, an imposed curse or punishment that might yet be set aright. We have spawned whole cultures of belief centered in the conviction that death is an illusion, is not our final fate, perhaps is only a preliminary before real, eternal life ensues. Very little expression of such aspirations has been scientific, or even rational; most is deeply embedded in the unconscious or in myths or in religious traditions and practices. Yet surely one of the striking facts about contemporary life is that one can begin at least to speculate on the possibility that death is eliminable in an apparently rational and scientifically plausible fashion. Of course such speculation may be only a contemporary form of myth-making and sophisticated death denial, but before reaching any such critical conclusion the attempt rationally and scientifically to conceive of the death of death must be given its due.

Much of what follows will be cast in terms of what is empirically, scientifically possible, both theoretically and in developing practice. But that is misleading, for what I am essentially interested in here is not speculation about empirical and emerging technological possibilities, but rather conducting a *thought experiment* to discover whether there are circumstances under which endless life would be appealing. To be duly rational in these inquiries we must satisfy ourselves with answers to such philosophical and value-laden questions before proceeding to invest resources in the development of technologies that superficially appear beneficial but which might finally prove to be unbearably burdensome. By trying to think through what would be required to attain human immortality, what criteria such existence would need to satisfy in order to interest us, what the conditions and implications of such living are, we will be in a much better position to decide whether such life is worthwhile. Moreover, we might also hope to understand more profoundly the issue raised in chapter two, on whether death is an evil.

Causes of Aging

An early step in advancing our understanding of the prospects for potentially endless life would be a resolution of the raging debate among biologists over theories of aging. Do bodies become more decrepit as cells become less efficient at sustaining themselves (a) because of the accumulation of waste products never completely eliminated; or (b) because the DNA in reproducing itself gradually accumulates random errors; or (c) because some cells simply stop reproducing after reaching maturity, so that as they die various organs suffer diminished functional capacity? Or (d) is there a built-in clock that runs out after a limited number of cell reproductions (estimated by Leonard Hayflick to be about fifty)?[1] The resolution of this debate will not occur in the abstract; it will likely occur with the devising of a therapy capable of altering the biological processes of aging. Whether through chemotherapies or recombinant DNA, the discovery of technologies capable of slowing down or even completely arresting aging will be the scientific breakthrough that makes the expectation of immortality a reasonable one.

Beyond this monumental advance, we must of course count on the continued progress of medical research to discover the causes of disease and to develop vaccines and cures. Being able as well to stimulate the regeneration of damaged organs and limbs, or to replace them altogether, would be another essential element in making plausible hopes for immortality. With all this, then—the cessation of natural aging, preventions and cures for disease, therapies for regenerating or replacing damaged body parts—would we have finally achieved a capacity for immortality?

Not entirely. As impressive as such achievements are, they cannot guarantee that no one need ever die. As creatures of inevitably limited power and understanding, however enlarged our durability or capacities, we would still be subject to death by accident and willful violence. No degree of progress in biological sciences will enable us to restore bodies disintegrated in the most devastating accidents or incinerated in a nuclear holocaust.[2] But by eliminating "natural death," death through the biological processes of aging, decline, disease, and demise, we would have so restricted the causes of human death that we could plausibly speak of attaining immortality.

Forms of Immortality

It is certainly the case that such speculations as the preceding are in a vein highly atypical of most reflections on immortality. Most who have considered eternal or near eternal life have thought about it not in terms of present life continuing indefinitely, but rather of a life *subsequent* to this one, in a different domain of existence. Ponce de Leon and his clones aside, most speculation has been about human beings living after death, not about human beings never dying. Such renewed life has been imagined to take a wide variety of forms, the chief of which seem to be (a) rebirth and reincarnation; (b) personal survival as a disembodied, "nonmaterial" soul or spirit; and (c) a re-created, resurrected bodily existence. (I count here only clearly personal or individual survivals, not worlds in which individual consciousness merges into group consciousness or some cosmic unity. The reason for this restriction will be explained presently.)

But I think the only fully rational speculation of the possibility of immortality must be along the scientific lines earlier considered. With the other forms of alleged immortality it is possible to be fairly brief. Any version of ongoing life proposed to our consideration--scientific, religious, psychological, whatever--would have to meet three major criteria if any particular individual is to have an interest in attaining such life: it must be personal survival, it must be believable, and it must be desirable.

Criteria for Worthwhile Survival

If the alleged form of survival is not personal—if that which continues is not identifiable as me, does not have my memories, consciousness, sensibilities, or other crucial attributes—it is difficult to understand in what sense it is I who survives at all, rather than merely some part of my former self. My hair may survive my death indefinitely as a wig for another, but no one would be seriously tempted to suggest that I therefore have survived. More than merely some part of my body must continue; most essentially, my unique consciousness must endure if we are to be

at all inclined to say that I survive death. It is for this reason that all notions of consciousness merging into a cosmic unity are disqualified as candidates for plausible notions of immortality. Similarly, my survival in the
memories of *others* will not be the sort of immortality that counts as
fully personal, however much fame might otherwise be desirable.

As for the other criteria that an acceptable notion of immortality must
satisfy, they are straightforward. To be believable, a hypothesis must be coherent, consistent, and supported by good reasons. It meets these requirements if it is free of internal contradictions, compatible with other beliefs, and backed by evidence that goes beyond mere intuition and
vague feeling. To be desirable, our notion of immortality must be one in
which the conditions of continuing life are at least tolerable, and prefera-
bly highly beneficial. Any notion of ongoing life that fails to be either personal, believable, or desirable will be unacceptable.

Applying the Criteria

The first notion of immortality above—that of rebirth or reincarnation,
perhaps as a member of a different species—fails to appeal precisely because it is a puzzle how *I* can be said to survive when in fact all that continues is a set of serial selves mysteriously connected one to another. Physical continuity, even contiguity in time, is absent in some versions (it
may be some considerable time before "I" reappear); continuity of species-
identity is absent ("I" could return as a wallaby) and usually there is no
(conscious) memory connection alleged.[3] In all these ways, notions of reincarnation fail to satisfy the criterion of *personal* survival, and perhaps as
well that of being a *desirable* condition. It might be sufficient grounds for rejecting this form of immortality as desirable that even its advocates seem
most to look forward to the day when one achieves release from recur-
ring serial lives.[4]

The second notion of ongoing existence, as a disembodied soul, is, if
anything, even less appealing. In the first place, it rests upon the classic
dualism of mind and body as entirely distinct substances capable of existing apart, and in which only mental substance is essential to personal identity. But these notions, while central to modern philosophy, have been
broadly rejected and refuted by contemporary philosophers, and are
thus today not readily believable.[5]

Beyond this consensus among contemporary philosophers, a still better ground for rejecting this vision of continuing life is that the conditions under which one would live must be far from ideal. On reflection,
who really would choose a life wholly devoid of the possibility of sen-
sory and sensual experience, a life without sex, the satisfaction of physical hunger, the smell of a spring morning in the forest, seeing the sun
set on a lake in the evening, or hearing Beethoven's sublime *Eroica* Sym-
phony. How are we to suppose any of these perceptions to be possible

without the bodily sensations that give rise to them? Even the most avid enthusiast of intellectual pursuits has generally supposed that satisfactory living must involve more than simply thought. But what else is possible for a non bodily, non material mind, soul, or spirit? It is one of the ironies of our time that persons not even greatly taken with the peculiar pleasures of the contemplative life should look with eager anticipation to the day when nothing else is available to them as disembodied spirits! Hence I conclude that survival as a disembodied spirit, if even possible, would be undesirable.[6]

The orthodox, or at least *early*, Christian vision of an afterlife, *perhaps* eternal, in which, through the exercise of divine power, God re-creates individual persons cannot be so easily dismissed.[7] It suffers none of the obvious defects of the previously noted notions of immortality. It promises personal survival, has wide appeal, and has been widely believed, regardless of what difficulties may inhere in it. While physical continuity is necessarily absent (we must still die to this life in this world) and temporal contiguity is most likely missing (we must await the "day of judgment" before being re-created), nonetheless memory and a renewed network of social relationships tie together my present self with the divinely re-created and resurrected self. As an embodied creature, presumably with a new and vastly improved version of a body, I can continue to enjoy the satisfaction of sexual and other bodily pleasures, no doubt at higher levels than presently and without the all too frequent bitter aftertastes that now afflict us.[8]

Because afterlife is envisioned as bodily, this conception of possible immortality escapes the objections to dualism that apply to the survival of mere "souls"; because the bodies we will supposedly have are improved versions of our present bodies, fully capable of experiencing all the pleasurable sensations earlier known to us, and more, it escapes the objection that the loss of bodily sensations is too severe to make such life desirable; and because such re-created bodily selves will satisfy both physical and mental criteria for identifying and reidentifying a person as the same person, we may suppose there is no concern here that such an afterlife is not personal. But for all this, the view that we shall survive as re-created and resurrected embodied persons does not entirely escape objections to its believability.

It is not fundamentally difficult to believe that God can and will resurrect humans, create the world anew, provide us with improved bodies, conquer all forms of evil, eliminate all burdensome scarcity, vanquish death, and so on. The fundamental difficulty is in believing that there exists, has ever existed, or will ever exist, or even could exist, such a Being as this. If we can believe in God the Creator, we can certainly believe in God the Re-Creator. But if the former view is not altogether believable, because it is not coherent, or because it is inconsistent with other of our beliefs, or because it is just not well supported by analysis, argument, and evidence, then surely the latter view is still less plausible.

Endless Life on Earth

It would be as inappropriate here to veer off on a refutation of theism or a defense of atheism as it was earlier to refute dualism. For the sake of continuing this thought experiment on immortality, I will not attend further to notions of afterlife, of re-created or disembodied selves, but will instead consider only the scenerio in which human beings cease dying of "natural" causes. Hence we are back to the possibility that some combination of genetic engineering, chemotherapies, and organ regeneration or replacement might be so successful as to prolong life indefinitely into the future, so far in fact that we could reasonably speak of human immortality.

I have already argued that this conception of immortality is believable, because it is consistent with what we know of biological processes—or, perhaps more accurately, what we do not know but are likely to learn in the near future—and the developing capacity of humans to manipulate those processes. More than any other view of immortality, this view most likely guarantees that the person who endures remains the same person. For here alone do we have uninterrupted continuity in space and time, and the likelihood of unifying memory as well. But the third criterion that needs to be satisfied before endorsing this view of immortality is desirability, and the desirability of unending continuation of life, even without fear of the ravages of aging, is extremely difficult to determine. The main task for the rest of this chapter is to explore just this issue.

When we try to think of what it might be like for life to continue indefinitely, potentially endlessly, three possibilities occur. We might suppose that only a single, unique individual is possessed of the capacity for endless life. This is playwright Karel Capek's speculation in *The Makropulos Secret*. In that work we meet Emilie Marty (a.k.a. Elina Makropulos, a.k.a. any number of other predecessors, all with "E.M." as initials), who, when we meet her, is 339 years old—or rather, more accurately, has been 39 for 300 years. Her youthfulness is preserved by an elixir, discovered by her father, that will presumably continue to work so long as she takes it.

Or, on the other hand, we might suppose a universal immortality, in which, say, some permanent alteration in human genetic structures and the mechanisms of cell nurturance and reproduction allows continuous individual life. To contemplate this possibility, we must imagine far more than how the conditions of living indefinitely change the terms of life for a single individual. Instead, we must anticipate radical social transformations, perhaps even changes in what we are prepared to call "human nature." The enormous imaginative leaps requisite to trying to conceive of human social life without individual death are what makes this a popular theme for science fiction writers.

Finally, between the possibility of a unique individual being immortal and everyone being so, there is the supposition of the survival of a select few. This elite of immortals could be created through either random mutagenesis or social selection and conferral. Genetic mutation is the mechanism imagined by Jonathan Swift to bestow immortality upon the Struldburgs, and in the early musings of Gulliver—before he actually meets these pitiful creatures—Gulliver imagines them to be possessed of rare wisdom and perspicacity, wealth, power, and peacefulness. Social selection and conferral, however, produce the more likely scenerario if indefinite longevity is to be attained by means of newly developed medical technologies.

However extensive we imagine this immortality to be—whether it is possessed by but one person, universally participated in, or shared by a select few—it is vital to require that it not be the cursed immortality suffered by the Struldburgs. For while these pitiable people never died a natural death, neither did they cease aging. Theirs was a fate of suffering ever deeper disability, enfeeblement, and disconnection from others. So it is essential to remember that no matter how extensively immortality is spread about, a minimum necessary condition for any form of it to be desirable is that both death and aging, after the attainment of a suitable age, be eliminated, and that undiminished vitality last as long as life itself.

Evaluating any of these possibilities as a desirable condition for anyone is a difficult venture, for much is left to imaginative speculation. Moreover, the kinds of difficulties that can be plausibly envisioned for each are substantially different, even different in kind, ranging from concerns about personal boredom to considerations of social justice. In the end, however, it seems to me not at all likely that prolonged survival, as a single individual, or as one member of an immortal species, or as one member of an elite group selected for indefinite longevity, is clearly in an individual's interest. This then presents a very puzzling paradox, for as I argued in chapter two, death is not a good thing. Now it may appear that neither dying nor indefinitely continuous living is a desirable state for human beings. Such a paradox raises a whole new set of questions.

Endless Life for All

Consider first the universal attainment of immortality for all of humanity. Either this would happen all at once, through some immediate alteration in everyone's genetic structures, or it would occur somewhat more gradually. In either case, the consequences seem unlikely to be beneficial. Ironically, an immediate conferral of universal immortality would seem, most likely, to lead to the destruction of humanity. Clearly a world suddenly populated by persons who did not die would radically alter every existing economic system. Such a shock to economic systems can be reasonably supposed to bring about revolution, territorial warfare, or at least massive social upheaval. In today's world, dominated by economies that have attained the capacity to destroy everything, it would be reasonable to suppose that the end of natural death would be so disruptive as to invoke the onslaught of violent death. This would seem all the more likely if reproduction of the species were not completely curtailed—and there is no reason to suppose that simply because people stopped dying they would stop populating. On the contrary!

But suppose the acquisition of immortality were phased in gradually, although still universally. Would this assure continuation of the species? No, but it might seem at least more likely to preserve the species over the short run. One of the first things that would have to change, however, is the continued reproduction of the species. Very early the carrying capacity of the earth could be exceeded, and the only way to assure the survival of existing humans would minimally be to require an end to reproduction.

What the consequences of a static, essentially unchanging population would be for the species and for each individual is scarcely imaginable. When two of T.S. Eliot's trilogy of basic facts, birth and death, have been largely eliminated from human experience, there is no predicting the impact upon culture and individual lives. And while we cannot say with certainty that lives lived with only copulation available as a central experience would not be worthwhile or meaningful, surely a large degree of skepticism is warranted.

The requirement for assuring that endless life for everyone would be advantageous and desirable is that in addition to eliminating natural death we would have to eliminate nearly all other restrictions as well. It is not possible to think very long of how life without natural death would be tolerable without also being prepared to think of human beings with unlimited intellect and understanding, unlimited natural resources of all sorts necessary to sustain life, unlimited goodwill to make continued community and peace between communities possible, and so on.

A case in point, illustrative of the claim that to eliminate death forces one to eliminate many other limits, is Alvin Silverstein's *Conquest of Death*.[9] Among the many utopian speculations in which Silverstein indulges are the following, all somehow supposed to be social consequences of the biological conquest of death: drunken driving is legislated off the road, and war itself becomes unthinkable, because life becomes "immeasurably valuable" (208); crime will be vastly diminished by cheap, effective, and safe mood-altering drugs that eliminate motivation for violence (210–211); learning will be easier and faster through the use of "knowledge pills" (211). And so on.

Silverstein's general strategy is to assume that what must occur to make social life possible once death is eliminated will occur. And this, of course, is the most blatant sort of Pollyanish utopian thinking imaginable. But as fantastic as these sorts of speculations may be, there is no escaping them if we are to conceive how universal immortality could be a desirable condition. It is clear that attempts to conceive of human beings as immortal require an ambitious exercise of utopian thinking. And to the degree that the latter is naive or simplistic, implausible and even undesirable, so too is the positing of universal human immortality. If these utopian speculations strike one as silly or misbegotten, then we must think as well that universal immortality is not an attractive possibility, for the species or for individual human beings.[10]

Endless Life for
One Person Only

Far down the scale from positing immortality for all is to restrict its conferral to but a single individual. In asking whether this would be a desirable condition for the person so endowed, we face a far different set of considerations. Our concerns now are not at the level of whether society itself can survive, but rather whether a single individual bestowed with the capacity for endless life can maintain a coherent identity and find such living worthwhile. Contrary to the impression that may have been conveyed in an earlier chapter, I do think this a very serious problem.

Bernard Williams worries that an individual living endlessly would encounter numerous serious problems. Among these are (1) intolerable tedium, boredom, and ennui as "categorical desire" necessarily wanes; (2) difficulties in sustaining a single identity, rather than an endless array of serial selves; and (3) the deadness of soul born of a meaningless existence that ensues as all human relationships prove to be temporary and fleeting. Earlier I considered only the first problem listed above, and I dismissed it as implausible, since the world is so varied and offers endless opportunities for growth and challenge, and I claimed further that mere repetition of experience is no reason to think life would become boring. This is true whether we are considering one, some, or all persons as immortal. However, where only one person in all the world is to be supposed immortal, Williams's fears of sustaining personal identity and of meaninglessness are much more substantial. And Williams does clearly have in mind the Makropulos case, in which a single individual potentially lives forever.

The difficulty in sustaining a single identity through endless existence lies in the continuously changing historical circumstances, experiences, and relationships of the person who never dies. So varied would these be over the long course of events that presumably the psychological states of an immortal being would also change substantially enough to warrant our regarding this not as one person in continuous existence but rather as a series of distinct selves in one body. The single most important factor in preventing continuity of identity is the alleged impossibility of any single person's sustaining categorical desire indefinitely. If continuity of identity is impossible, then continued existence clearly cannot be of much interest to one who will not continue as a single identifiable self but rather as an endless series of selves.

But I have argued in chapter two that there is insufficient reason to believe that categorical desire will necessarily wane for humans over an endless life-span. The most important of our (categorical) desires are linked to renewable appetites, and hence are not so ephemeral as Williams fears. This being so, there is similarly little reason to believe that continuity of identity cannot be sustained. The fear, therefore, that endless life would require discontinuous serial selves is unwarranted. Thus, finally, it cannot be supposed that endless life for any individual is undesirable because no one *could* endure as a single self through an indefinite future.

Williams's final reservation about the desirability of endless life is the most troubling. In the situation in which one person lives indefinitely, and no one else does, insuperable barriers to sustaining the kinds of human relationships that make life worthwhile and meaningful arise. Of necessity, relations between an immortal person and everyone else are, from the point of view of the immortal, temporary and relatively brief. For one who never dies, sustaining intimacy and openness with those who do die could prove impossible. It is here, rather than in the demise of categorical desire as such, that the greatest difficulty in sustaining a coherent identity is likely to arise. And it is here as well that the most severe challenge to endless life being worthwhile is to be found. It is reasonable to suppose that where the maintenance of deep and sustaining human relationships is impossible, a life that continues endlessly would be one worthy only of Dante's innermost circle of Hell.

But it is by no means certain that sustaining human relationships are impossible for the sole immortal being we are hypothesizing. After all, it might be objected, even in our finite, mortal lives most of us suffer severe losses through death, departures, or divorce. We change schools, jobs, and communities; grandparents, parents, spouses, and even children die; divorce is frequent; and through it all, we go on. Some even thrive on frequent change, and would find life terminally dull if there were too much stability and too little variation.

This is not to deny that deep, secure human relationships are necessary for life to be meaningful over the long run, perhaps especially over the potentially infinite long run. It is only to point out that such relationships need not themselves be of infinite duration to be sustaining, so that one whose life did not end might still find deep human relations possible and worthwhile on a serial basis.

Despite all this, the wiser course would seem to be profound skepticism about the possibility of individual endless life being desirable. Even fifty-year relationships might come to seem like one-night stands to an immortal. Or alternatively, the cumulative burden of every intimate relationship ending in the death of the other might prove an overwhelming grief for an immortal. We cannot know, nor even speculate very well, since the main parameters within which human psychology presently operates—our finiteness, our mortality—are by hypothesis dissolved. Only the grounds for profound skepticism about the desirability of individual endless life are certain.

Endless Life for Some

It is as difficult, therefore, to suppose that being a single individual living endlessly would be any more in one's interest than being one member of an immortal species. Neither condition seems certain to provide the combination of circumstances that would allow such living to be simultaneously personal, believable, and desirable. This being so, we are left for contemplation only the supposition that one might live on as one of a group of select individuals upon whom immortality is bestowed.

In this final scenario there is much to be said for immortality, or at least there is less to be said against it. There is no reason to fear the immediate catastrophic social consequences likely when endless life is universally conferred, and little reason to suppose that even over the long run endless human life would be rendered impossible or meaningless. For members of the privileged elite of immortals, there is the prospect of ongoing community that allows for sustaining durable, intimate relationships. Thus as long as the capacity for desiring goods as ends in themselves remains viable, life remains healthy, and material conditions remain adequate, there is assured opportunity for finding endless life beneficial. For a specific individual thus possessed of immortality, there is much reason to believe immortality would be desirable.

From almost any other point of view than that of the egoistic rationality of one so privileged as to be immortal, there is much to be said against this form of deathlessness for a select group of individuals. What is chiefly to be said against it is simply that it is the rankest sort of social injustice. On what conceivable grounds could we fairly distribute the perhaps incomparable benefit of endless life? There is such a vast disparity between those receiving such a gift and all others that it is impossible to imagine what criteria could be used to identify some among us as deserving of endless life or what the compensating benefits for mortals left behind would be. And even supposing we could, in theory, solve the problem of a just distribution of such a precious good as immortality, who among us would suppose that an ideal solution would be implemented?

Human beings, it might be said, have always had to contend with unjust distributions of goods. Yet we have had as well the dour satisfaction of knowing that specific beneficiaries of injustice would suffer in the due course of time the same fate as those unjustly exploited for the comfort of the privileged. Now even this small consolation may be destroyed! The reification of inequality that conferring immortality upon an elite would engender exceeds all other injustices perpetrated by humankind, and would seem to do so in perpetuity.

It is to be wondered as well whether committing society to such a deeply embedded stratification would be genuinely in the eternal interest of even a seemingly privileged elite. What I have in mind here is not quite Plato's question of whether anything can be genuinely good for an individual that is not also in the common good. That question, I think, has been answered affirmatively by the long history of class society that has amply demonstrated just how well a few can live at the expense of the many. Rather, the question now must be whether the conditions of life for the privileged few who would live endlessly at the expense of the many are such that the very specific requirements for meaningful existence we have been considering can be satisfied.

In the relatively short run of a "natural" life-span, elites have fared very well indeed. But what we have discovered to be most essential to making infinite life worthwhile has been the opportunity and ability to sustain essentially human relationships of openness and intimacy. On this score, elites have not been notably successful throughout history. There is no good reason to suppose they would become so throughout eternity. There is then little reason to think that in fact, if not in principle, eternal life for one who is a member of a select group of immortals would really be desirable. For example, just one of the common pleasures of ordinary mortals that may become unavailable to immortals is the bearing and raising of children. Such children themselves might or might not be immortal. If not, their parents would suffer the agonies of seeing their offspring grow "older" than themselves and die. And if these children too have immortality bestowed upon them, we eventually encounter the difficulties that arise when everyone is immortal.

It must be confessed that these are relatively weak arguments against the suppostion that eternal life would be a good for one who was a member of an elite of immortals. All I have been able to say against this is that such a condition would be unjust and it might be difficult to maintain the sorts of relationships that could conceivably make such life worth continuing. But neither of these considerations counts decisively against the claim that life would be worthwhile for the deathless individual. While such life may not be morally desirable, it could, nonetheless, just like the lives of the most privileged now, be personally very attractive. What then should we conclude from this extended inquiry into the possible good of endless life?

Conclusions

First of all, we cannot conclude that endless life is certainly not desirable for one who receives it. Given the exactly right combination of circumstances and opportunities, it may well be. This in turn means that the paradox that death is a loss and endless life no gain is not as dramatic as feared. At worst it must be cast in terms of supposing that while death is certainly a loss for one, the attainment of immortality is at best a dubious gain. One with sufficiently dulled moral sensibilities may still hope that continuous life as one of a small elite of immortals would be satisfying and meaningful. There is no assurance that this is so, some reason to think not, and much moral objection to it. Nonetheless, the possibility is real enough to nurture an age-old hope.

Secondly, there is an eminently practical implication to be derived from this thought experiment. As far as justice is concerned, it would seem far preferable to commit our resources elsewhere than to research and technologies that might lead to a greatly prolonged life span. In particular, it would appear to be far more advisable to devote effort to assuring more people the opportunity to live out what is presently a "natural" life-span than to seek to prolong endlessly the lives of a few. And, it would be far better to use our resources and direct our research to improving the quality of life of the greater number of persons who will enjoy a full life-span. Even from the point of view of the beneficiaries of a potentially endless life this might be a preferable choice, given that such a prolonged life is at best a dubious good.[11]

The third conclusion, a theoretical one, is perhaps the most appropriate for such a hypothetical inquiry as this has been. It may be that the most profound insight into inquiring about the evil of death and the good of endless life is not that either of these can be known. Instead, it may strike one that the real import of all this is that human life is irremediably tragic. As finite and embodied creatures, we aspire to be more. Our fondest hopes for more, expressed as a desire to live endlessly, turn out to be a hope for a life that is unlikely to be very satisfying. Our greatest fear, the fear of annihilation, is almost certainly one that will, for each of us, be realized. We are left only with the prospect of four score and five years, if fortunate, and the struggle to make these meaningful years. For all of us, having this much life and the requisite opportunities to realize value in life requires enormous good fortune and some effort. But beyond this, in our hopes for more than this, the Fates themselves are in control and not we. And in that loss of ultimate control, in that final impotence, resides the tragedy inherent in human lives. We shall none of us escape this tragedy whatever the illusions we subscribe to in seeking to ward it off.

IV

FEARING DEATH AND CARING FOR THE DYING

> Now death is the most terrible of all
> things; for it is the end, and nothing is
> thought to be either good or bad for the
> dead . . . The brave man is as dauntless as
> man may be. Therefore, while he will fear
> even the things that are not beyond human
> strength, he will face them as he ought
> and as the rule directs, for honor's sake;
> for this is the end of virtue.
>
> Aristotle
> *Nichomachean Ethics*

Much is sometimes made of the fact that practicing physicians have a far greater fear of death than most persons, even greater than that of their dying patients. That this is so, I think, is widely believed on the basis of personal experience, anecdotes, and cultural stereotypes (e.g., Dr. Emerson in "Whose Life Is It Anyway?"), and is substantiated in at least one often cited psychological study by Herman Feifel. But what precisely can be properly concluded from this fact? Feifel, for his part, says this:

> There is the implication that a number of physicians utilize the medical profession, through which the individual secures prominent mastery over disease, to help control personal concerns about death. Nevertheless, in those instances where the physician's professional narcissism comes under attack–particularly in encounter with the fatally ill–his reawakened anxieties about death may lead him to unwittingly disinherit his patient psychologically at the very time he enhances attention to his physiological needs . . . Increased psychological kinship with the idea of oncoming death . . . would enhance emotional support for the physician and further maximize treatment of his patient.[1]

And Sally Gadow, noting Feifel's study and lamenting the unfortunate view that "death is one of life's greatest evils," which so many health professionals seem to hold, remarks, parenthetically, that "one might wish that health professionals, of all people, would have resolved for them-

selves such a profound difficulty in order to be of help to those who depend on that help in their dying."[2]

There is an association alleged here, in both Feifel and Gadow and
doubtless elsewhere as well,[3] between fear of death and suitability to
care for the dying. It is an association that for some borders on being a truism. The view seems to be that the more one fears death (or suffers
"death anxiety") the less able one is to meet the distinctive emotional
and psychological needs of the dying. But if we examine with some care
what is involved in such suppositions, it turns out that they (1) are far
more complex than they initially appear, (2) raise some very profound philosophical and conceptual problems, (3) are laden with highly conten-
tious normative moral notions, and (4) rely upon some very dubious
empirical-psychological theses. In trying to substantiate these claims, I
shall begin by constructing an argument that I trust fairly and rigorously
makes explicit what is suppressed in the reasoning that leads from an empirical finding of high death anxiety in physicians to the normative judgment that such persons ill serve their patients in important ways.

Consider the following attempt to unpack what is being both said and
implied above:

1. "Fear of death" and "death anxiety" are synonymous and inter-
changeable terms for the same phenomenon.

2. Death anxiety is a psychological phenomenon. It is regarded by
Weisman, for instance, as an aspect of "annihilation anxiety," as "a
dread of complete extinction, anxiety about becoming nothing at
all."[4]

3. Death anxiety leads necessarily to death denial–a psychological phenomenon whereby one seeks to deny one's own personal mortality.

4. The connection between death anxiety and death denial is either:
   a. psychologically well founded, or
   b. logical (a relation of identity); *i.e.*, to be anxious about death is to
   deny one's mortality, and to deny one's mortality is to be anxious
   about death.

5. Death denial is irrational (or at least nonrational): there are no compelling good reasons to fear death.

6. Death anxiety or death denial can be overcome by, for example,
maintaining open and honest relations with oneself and with others, or, in more serious cases, by the acquisition of self-knowledge
through a therapy that helps in countering such psychological defense mechanisms as isolation, dissociation, and the like.

7. Death denial (and hence death anxiety) makes one psychologically unfit to be of assistance to others who may be struggling to come to grips with their own dying. A physician, for example, may, in Feifel's words, "unwittingly disinherit his patient psychologically at the very time he enhances attention to his physiological needs."

8. Overcoming death denial and accepting death non-anxiously is a good thing and a desirable end for all to seek.

9. Hence, overcoming death anxiety and accepting one's mortality is a good thing for both health professionals and dying patients.

10. Therefore, health professionals who have not mastered their fear of death and death denial will not be capable of providing the kind of care that is maximally beneficial to dying patients.

In the following analysis of the above argument, I shall not take issue with the claim that physicians tend to have a higher than (statistically) normal fear of death. I shall raise some question about what this means, but once its meaning is clarified I will not challenge the empirical foundations of the claim. My chief effort is to show how tenuous is the connection between this claim and the conclusion that persons with such fears are ill suited to treat the dying. Indeed, in the end, I shall try to turn this connection on its head and argue that without self-conscious and intense awareness of one's own fear of death, one is unlikely to be of help to the dying. But before arriving at this initially implausible conclusion, it will be necessary to examine several kinds of issues raised by the intermediary steps of the above argument. As we proceed, it will be seen that these issues are frequently abstract and difficult. Nonetheless, they cannot be ignored if justice is to be done to the argument.

The first issue is raised in the second premise, and that has to do with the nature of death anxiety. The question here is whether death anxiety is simply a psychological phenomenon or whether it can be more broadly conceived as also (not alternatively) an ontological condition of the species. By this latter I mean nothing more grandiose than the supposition that some degree of fearing death may be intrinsic to human nature, or, better, to the human condition. If we understand human beings as creatures seemingly uniquely possessed, at least among beings known to us, of both self-consciousness and awareness of an external world, we already have taken the first step in positing death anxiety as fundamental to the human condition. And if next we suppose that this kind of consciousness is a transcendent consciousness, we may have enough to ground death anxiety ontologically.[5]

"Transcendent consciousness" here means the power possessed by human faculties of thinking, imagining, desiring, and the like to go beyond the natural limitations of human existence: the power, for instance, to know we shall die and to want to live on, to recognize the finiteness of our existence as a natural species in this world and to conceive of a divine order without such limitations, to live as all beings known to us do, as embodied beings, and to believe that we could live on eternally as disembodied souls.

No such beliefs, desires, or imaginings need be true for consciousness to be transcendent; they need only be possible, and we know that they are this. Death anxiety will be the accompaniment of such consciousness, precisely because it is the expression of the tension between our actual condition as finite and limited beings and our aspirations to be unlimited, immortal beings that a transcendent consciousness provides. Thus, the way out of ontologically grounded death anxiety is to eliminate transcendent consciousness, which is no less than to cease to be human, or to die. So understood, death anxiety is better than any of its alternatives! And finally, it is this (metaphysical) reality about the human condition, this ontological given of a transcendent consciousness in a finite being, that underlies the psychological phenomenon of death anxiety.

But if we do consider death anxiety simply as a psychological phenomenon, it can be readily seen how it is closely tied to death denial. Anxiety as a state of discomfort naturally leads to avoidance behavior. If one is anxious about death, this anxiety will be manifested in a reluctance to talk about death, think about it, or be in its presence (funerals, dying persons, etc.). The more pronounced forms of such avoidance behavior constitute death denial, the concerted attempt to shield oneself from all familiarity with death, especially reminders of one's own mortality. It is tempting, thus, to think of death anxiety and death denial as located at different points on the same continuum; but as death anxiety escalates, it merges with death denial until an identity of psychological states is achieved. Thus severe death anxiety constitutes denial, and death denial is severe death anxiety.

To succeed in its strongest form, the argument as originally cast needs this identity. Without it the case for supposing that those with higher than normal death anxiety are ill suited to care for the dying is greatly diminished. But the connection is not all that persuasive, and this for reasons other than that death anxiety is not simply a psychological phenomenon. It is plausible to suppose that death anxiety (*qua* psychological phenomenon) and death denial are identical only if we suppose that anxiety/denial on the one hand and death acceptance on the other are mutually exclusive extreme opposites, and that these two polar opposites exhaustively characterize possible responses to confronting one's own death. Both these suppositions are false.

The first claim–that death anxiety and death acceptance are mutually exclusive responses to death–is false simply as an empirical matter. Being anxious about death no more entails that one cannot make his or her accommodation to it than that making accommodation requires an absence of death anxiety. Psychological studies have shown the non-exclusivity of these two responses to death. Ray and Najman have shown that a more sophisticated scale for measuring the presence of death anxiety, in a range of attitudes toward death conceptually broader than is usually allowed for, reveals that "the assumption by Swenson and others[6] that death acceptance is the categorical opposite of death anxiety [is] false." Ray and Najman found some degree of death anxiety in the whole spectrum of responses to death.[7]

Of course in making such a discovery, a more profound error in the claim under examination is revealed, and that is its conceptual impoverishment. For supposing death anxiety to be identical with death denial makes it logically incompatible with any response to death except denial. But in fact, death anxiety is an element of each of the possible predominant strategies that, either through psychological compulsion or through free choice, a person may use in confronting death. I have argued in chapter one that in facing our own death (or another's) the general strategies employed are best characterized as denial, acceptance, and rebellion. Moreover, none of these is reducible to a psychological state. If this is so, the second claim needed to make the identity of death anxiety and death denial plausible—that denial and acceptance exhaustively characterize the alternatives available to us—is also undercut. But more important, if we think rather of death anxiety as fundamental, perhaps inescapable, and as an element in any approach to death, I believe we shall be able to think about and understand the issues here much more clearly.

We have now two reasons, one psychological, one ontological, for thinking death anxiety or the fear of death (still here used interchangeably) not so untoward a condition as the argument under examination supposes. There is a third, and to my mind, still stronger reason for not regarding such a fear so negatively, and that is that it may be entirely rational. The argument we are considering asserts, in premise five, that the fear of death is not rational, and goes on to use this conviction in suggesting, therefore, that such fear ought to be excised and that only if excised can one attain the desirable goals of accepting death for oneself and be of assistance to others in aiding them to accept death.

But how ought we to regard this basic assumption that the fear of death is not rational? The question here is most fundamentally one of whether it is correct to regard death as an evil, as a significant personal misfortune. For if it is an evil, in this sense clearly it will be reasonable to fear it, while if it is not correctly so regarded, fear will be misplaced. An exploration of the question "Is death an evil?" was undertaken in chapter two, but two remarks are in order here. The first is that for most people throughout history, worries about whether death is an evil and properly to be feared would be exceedingly strange: the popular wisdom has always been that of course death is fearful, evil, and something to be avoided. It would take powerful evidence to overturn so deep-seated a conviction and all of the cultural and religious practices predicated upon it.

Secondly, if one is not persuaded by appeal to tradition, culture, and religious heritage, there is available a straightforward secular and rational argument to the end that death is a great personal misfortune. The main line of argument in chapter two noted that death is not an evil for any features it has, it is an evil because life is good and death is the deprivation of just that good. Death is an evil because it is the irrevocable loss of opportunity, of possibility, of the continued good of life. Death is a deprivation of life; were one not dead, one would be alive, and his or her possibilities for satisfying experiences could be realized.

We have now several reasons for supposing death anxiety is not so untoward as the argument we set out initially to examine supposes. The first is that insofar as death anxiety is not identical with death denial, it is incorrect to regard anxiety as such as incompatible with giving the best care possible to the dying. While it may be true that a strong tendency to engage in death denial will render one ill-suited to care for the dying, death anxiety as such does not do so. Moreover, death anxiety may be inescapable, if indeed it is a necessary feature of the psychological makeup of finite beings with self-consciousness and not necessarily finite aspirations. Thus it is futile to regard a personal fear of death as incompatible with optimal care of the dying, since "optimal care" or the "best possible care" must, by definition, be compatible with what humans are capable of doing. Finally, there is good reason to believe that some degree of fearing death is a well-founded and entirely reasonable response to reflecting on absolute annihilation.

For all these reasons, it seems to me that the proper way to regard the relation of death anxiety to a capacity to give the best possible care to dying persons is quite other than the argument we have been considering supposes. Rather than regarding the fear of death as incompatible with good care for the dying, it seems more correct that we regard it as a necessary component of giving such care. We should not seek to "overcome," "master," or "control" such a fear. Nor, of course, should we seek, as a general rule, to enhance such fears, or be mastered or controlled by them. Instead, the wiser course would seem to be to acknowledge them for what they are: real, inescapable, reasonable. And with a heightened sensitivity to and awareness of this aspect of our (psychological, ontological, and rational) makeup, we can deal with such fear as openly and as honestly as possible.

Such a recommendation for how best to deal with feelings often thought incompatible with right living (or dying) is by no means unprecedented or even unfamiliar. Consider just one analogical situation, that of certain forms of sexual attraction. It is well established by now that between parents and children living together there will be inevitably very powerful and explicit sexual feelings. There is compelling reason in human society not to encourage the acting out of these powerful feelings. Yet, at the same time, we have learned that repression or attempts at exorcism do not succeed in eliminating such attractions, and that on

the contrary both such strategies have had highly deleterious consequences. The most viable course has seemed to be the candid acknowledgment, at least on the part of self-aware and sensitive adults, of these feelings. Exactly what social form such acknowledgment ought to take is no
doubt a matter of constant and continuing controversy. But at least recognizing the reality and the power of these feelings to oneself, *qua* child,
qua parent, seems to do much to diminish their threat (and the temptation to act on them). And so similarly it may be with the fear of death.

Many of the points I have sought to make in the foregoing in response to contemporary beliefs were made more elegantly and incisively
by Aristotle twenty-four centuries ago. In his analysis of the virtue of courage, Aristotle considers whether the courageous person is ever afraid.
About this he has different things to say, but his essential position
would seem to be that fear of death, in the right proportion, for the
right reason, at the right time, is altogether compatible with courage. Indeed, one who is utterly fearless before death is foolish perhaps to the
point of madness, and one who is sanguine to that which really is terrible is rash. But the brave person is genuinely concerned with what is
most terrible:

> No man is more likely than he to stand his ground against what is awe-
> inspiring. Now death is the most terrible of all things; for it is the end,
> and nothing is thought to be either good or bad for the dead. . . . The
> brave man is as dauntless as man may be. Therefore, while he will fear
> even the things that are not beyond human strength, he will face them
> as he ought and as the rule directs, for honor's sake; for this is the end
> of virtue.[8]

Aristotle thus recognizes death as an evil, sees that fear is inescapable
for human beings, and nonetheless believes that such fear is compatible
with a courageous response to annihilation, and not merely compatible
but, to the degree its absence is mad or rash, desirable and reasonable.
And such courage, surely, is part of any defensible view of how death
should best be accommodated.

After all this, can I claim to have shown that the initial allegation associ-
ating high death anxiety with diminished capacity for extending opti-
mum care to the dying is mistaken? Not at all! But what truth there is in
such allegations must be attained through considerable clarification and
far more careful articulation. In light of the foregoing discussion, I believe we capture the essential truths best by recasting the reasoning as follows:

1. "Death anxiety" designates that psychological phenomenon that
consists in feeling dread of complete annihilation. "Fear of death" is
a belief that death is frightening, and a belief that may be more or
less reasonably supported.

2. Death anxiety is distinct from death denial, where the latter is a psychological phenomenon whereby one seeks to avoid confrontation with all reminders of one's own personal mortality. Anxiety about death is part of denial, just as it is present in psychologically more comfortable attitudes toward death, but it is not identical with any of these attitudes.

3. A high degree of death denial ill suits one to give optimal care to the dying, for suffering such unacknowledged anxiety leads one to avoid or "disinherit" someone whose situation is personally threatening to the death denier.

4. Severe death denial can be diminished by open and honest relations with oneself and with others, or, in more serious cases, by the acquisition of self-knowledge through a therapy that helps in countering such psychological defense mechanisms as isolation, dissociation, etc.

5. Some degree of death anxiety is inescapable and some degree of fear of death is desirable in human beings. Honest and open acknowledgments of the reality and presence of such feelings and beliefs are important attributes for those who would extend maximally beneficial assistance to the dying.

6. Therefore, without such recognition of one's own fears and feelings, health professionals cannot offer the best care to their terminally ill patients.

In closing, it is worth remarking on at least one large issue in the original argument that has not been directly engaged in this discussion, and that is the highly prescriptive notion that ultimately what we all ought to strive for is "to accept death." Such a notion is sometimes regarded as too obviously correct to warrant comment, and sometimes represented simply as an empirical given, a "psychologically adaptive attitude" to take toward death in which the implicit and controversial moral prescriptions on how we ought to live and die are simply assumed. It seems to me there are more or less defensible ways to formulate this notion of accepting death, and that the less defensible tend in the direction of equating accepting death with approving of death, with regarding death somehow as a good. But I have been vague and evasive on this issue because I think it is at least as large and murky and in need of careful consideration as are the notions of death anxiety, fear, and denial discussed here. And while I had some critical things to say of death acceptance in chapter one, far more attention needs to be paid to such notions as "good death," "natural death," "death with dignity," a "right to die," and the like. That, therefore, is the burden of the next two chapters.

V

IS A NATURAL DEATH
A GOOD DEATH?

> There is no such thing as a natural death:
> nothing that happens to a man is natural,
> since his presence calls the world into
> question. All men must die: but for every
> man his death is an accident and, even if
> he knows it, an unjustifiable violation.
>
> Simone de Beauvoir
> *A Very Easy Death*

Before proceeding directly with consideration of the immensely difficult (and obscure) question of whether a "natural" death is a "good" death, it might be helpful to summarize some of our findings so far. In the first chapter I argued that, broadly speaking, there were three approaches to one's own death that had been adopted by individual human beings. These were called denial, acceptance, and rebellion, and each was characterized as more than merely a psychological state but less than a fully developed philosophy. The analysis there showed that while each had certain strengths and weaknesses, there was the most to be said for rebellion against death. Rebellion was understood to be a commitment to affirming the value of each individual life,[1] and further, rebellion satisfied the conviction that only in resisting that which limits human possibilities for fulfillment and achievement could one realize his or her fullest humanity. Since chapter one, I have been trying to work out the implications of that position for a variety of concerns one might have about death, including whether death is an evil, whether death is the worst evil one might suffer, whether immortality would be good, whether it is rational to fear death, whether one who fears death can adequately take care of the dying, and so on.

In chapter two, I argued a fairly narrow thesis, that death was indeed always an evil, in that it was always, for the one who suffered it, the loss of all possibility of satisfying experience. One can, to be sure, suffer such loss without being dead, and this is perhaps even worse—if only because it so undermines human dignity. Nonetheless, it is death that does this for most of us, and, for every one of us, to suffer death is to suffer a great evil. Similarly, in chapter three we found abundant reason to be skeptical that immortality would be beneficial. It was important in those chapters, as it will be important in this one, to keep in mind that the point of view from which notions of good and bad death are being evaluated is a subjective one, one of rational egoism, and not one in which each of us conceives ourself as a "world-historical" figure, to use Kierkegaard's ironic phrase.

Chapter four argued the thesis that it was rational to fear death and followed out the implications of this in the practical realm of caring for the dying. It would perhaps be sufficient to show the rationality of fearing death by showing that death is an evil. Not resting content with this foundation, however, I suggested that the fear of death might have deeper roots in the human condition and thus not be avoidable. In any case, it did not seem to me to constitute a real barrier to providing good care to those with the special needs the terminally ill often have. Quite the contrary, a keen awareness of one's fear of death may well be an altogether necessary condition for meeting those needs in others.

In all that has preceded, a certain amount of "conceptual clarification" was necessary, as for instance in distinguishing the fear of death from death denial. Secondly, it was several times necessary to point out that important questions of value and morality were being begged, that some positions of considerable controversy were being assumed without benefit of supporting argument. This occurred, for instance, when, in chapter one, we found that some authors have simply assumed that a universally desirable goal is to bring every dying person to the "stage" where he or she "accepts" death. Third, we found occasions when the distinction between what is the case and what ought to be the case was confused. This occurred, to use the same example, when we found the "death counselor" sliding from a description of the last days of a person with terminal cancer to prescribing such (usual) behavior as correct and desirable. Clearly these sorts of errors overlap, and in the worst cases are all present. Talk about "natural death" and "good death" may well be just such a worst case.

The Uses of "Natural Death"
in Moral and Political Discourse

Consider for a moment the variety of uses to which some notion or other of "natural death" is implicitly being put when it is claimed that "A person has a right to a natural death with dignity." At least five different significant claims can be extracted from the assertion of this single sentence:

1. *A Right to Be Respected.* Either a moral or a legal right, or both, might be asserted here. Sometimes the moral right is said to be derivative from some more fundamental right, such as a right to self-determina-

tion or autonomy; sometimes it seems to be regarded as itself basic. Similarly, as a legal right, it might be supposed rooted in the Constitution, as derived from the well established Constitutional "right to privacy," or it might be thought to be founded on precedents established by court decisions. Increasingly, at the present time, attempts are being made to define legislatively, through statutory law, an explicit right to a natural death.[2]

2. *An Ideal to Be Achieved.* To die a "natural death" is sometimes thought to be the best way for one to exit the world. As such, it is more than a right to be respected, and becomes an ideal to be achieved. When "natural death" is linked with a notion of "human dignity," it acquires a moral stature it could not have alone. Among its most enthusiastic advocates, "natural death" almost seems to be a duty, and one is urged to "strive to die naturally." The romanticization of dying can even extend to the claim, against all reason, that death is "the final stage of growth" and a much to be desired achievement.

3. *A Guide to Medical Treatment.* Some notion of "natural death" is invoked to guide decision-making about when to institute or discontinue life-prolonging medical treatment. Sometimes the use of "artifical means" to sustain life is thought "unnatural" and "undignified," and physicians are urged "to let Nature take its course." In this vein as well, pneumonia has been called "the old man's friend,"—especially prior to the discovery and use of powerful antibiotics—because it sometimes kills those suffering a slow, debilitating dying "naturally" and prevents a prolongation of meaningless or dreadfully burdensome life.

4. *A Guide to Public Policy.* Given the foregoing uses of "natural death" as a right, an ideal, and a guide for medical decision making, it is only a slight further extension to use it as the inspiration for making public policy. As such, it will presumably help direct us in how to divide scarce health resources between life-prolonging technologies and making provision for the needs of the dying. Further, it will shape statutory law to give expression of our "rights," protect our "dignity," and allow for the attainment of our aspirations. All of this was sought in a single piece of legislation just over a decade ago, in the "California Natural Death Act." In that legislation Californians were accorded a "right" to discontinue "artificial" treatments that "undermined dignity" and prevented a "natural death."[3]

5. *An Argument for Accepting Death.* As we have already seen in the first three chapters, death as a fact of nature, as inevitable, inescapable, and necessary to organic systems, is regarded as "natural death" and is taken to be a reason for each of us to become sanguine in confronting death. Francis Bacon's famous dictum "It is as natural to die as it is to be born" is supposed to be not only obviously true, but a compelling reason for not resisting or rebelling against death.

These highly varied uses of the term "natural death" in moral and politi-

cal discourse are badly in need of critical evaluation. This evaluation, however, must of necessity await the prior task of seeking some clarification
of meaning for "natural death." It is a phrase that means many different
things, often in a single use. Thus it is vital in evaluating the truth of
such claims as are made above that we first have some better notion of precisely what each claim means.

The Meanings of "Natural"
as Applied to Death and Dying

There are any number of strategies for sorting out the various ways "natural" is used and how it applies to both death and dying. Dallas High[4]
has characterized seven different meanings, and Robert Veatch[5] five distinct senses; neither believes himself to have exhausted the possible applications of the term even to death and dying. Daniel Callahan,[6] pursuing
a different strategy, forsakes trying to make coherent the diversity of
uses of "natural" and elects instead to argue for the usefulness of a
stipulative and reformative definition of "natural death" that he believes
will bring clarity and provide guidance in the crucial areas of shaping public policy and allocating health resources between combating death and
providing services to the dying. The following division of discourse
using "natural" into six categories owes most to those of High and
Veatch, although it neither "splits the difference" between them nor entirely agrees with either at crucial junctures.

1. *Scientific* (Biological). The first and perhaps most familar use of "natural" characterizes as natural that which is in accord with laws descriptive
of the operations of the universe, i.e., of "nature." The laws of physics
are paradigmatic, but in the context that most interests us now, it is biological law, the principles characteristic of the functioning of organic systems, that makes death "natural." According to this use of "natural,"
such expressions as "Death is inevitable, unavoidable, and necessary
and thus natural" are readily intelligible. Here, strictly speaking, to act
contrary to nature is not possible. For anything that seems to violate natural law will be evidence only that we have not properly formulated or understood natural law, not that the phenomenon is genuinely an exception.

It is, indisputably, the nature of living organisms to die. By itself, however, the strictly scientific use of "natural" has no moral implications,
for from the fact that things happen according to this understanding of natural law, it follows neither that they ought or they ought not to do so. Indeed, such judgments are altogether inappropriate, as scientific natural
law purports merely to describe how natural systems do in fact operate;
it implies nothing about how we should judge these operations.

2. *Statistical.* In this sense, that which is "natural" is that which is in ac-

cord with statistical generalities, with what is the average or mean or median occurrence of the event. For example, for a woman born in the developed world to die at age 78 would in this sense be "natural," since the life expectancy of females born in the developed world is, statistically, 78. For such a woman to live to age 95 would be "unnatural," for it would be a significant deviation from the statistical norm. But here again, as with scientific law, what is "natural" or "unnatural" is entirely without moral implication. We cannot straightaway draw moral conclusions from what usually happens any more than we can from what invariably happens; in both cases we need intervening premises of a normative nature about what ought to be the case.

3. *Anthropological.* This is Veatch's term for a category of "natural" and "unnatural" that is defined almost entirely negatively. That which is, in this sense, "natural" is that which is not artificial, or not humanly made. Something is "natural" if found so in nature, untouched by human hands, processing, or artifice. Wood is natural, plastic is not. Cow's milk is natural; bacon laced with nitrites and other preservatives is not. It was easy to find the opposite of "natural" when considering scientific or statistical uses of the term; it is rather more difficult in the somewhat more nebulous category of the anthropological. Here far more is left to subjective judgment: is granola natural and Frosted Flakes unnatural? According to what criteria?

However more nebulous and subjective the category of the anthropologically natural may be, it is clear that like the foregoing, this use of "natural" does not allow for any straightforward value judgments either. To derive a general moral conclusion from a premise about what is (anthropologically) natural would require an intervening premise to the effect that anything artificial, processed, or humanly made is somehow bad. At the very least, such a sweeping premise would render far too much of life unacceptable to be palatable to most of us, and it is simply not a very persuasive notion.

4. *Conventional.* That which is "natural" is that which is familiar, unsurprising, and usual. This category closely resembles but is not identical with the statistical. It is different in that it is far more impressionistic and subjective, depending as it does upon individual or cultural variables in human experience. What is familiar and usual in our experience may have nothing to do with scientific law, little to do with statistical norms, and less still to do with human artifice; but it may have much to do with the peculiarities of the time, place, and environment we find ourselves in.

Most people in the late twentieth century United States are shocked and dismayed by the death of a young child. That is an unusual and unfamiliar event in our experience. It has, of course, not always been so, and for other people in other times and in other material conditions, the survival of infants to adulthood may have been unusual.

Be this as it may, it must be acknowledged that at least a great deal of what underlies many moral judgments is just such conventionality. We are prone to judge as morally untoward that which is not customary and not known to us. Much of what we count as morality is largely a matter of conventionality, and even that part of morality that has a significant critical component is arrived at through sensibilities conditioned by the peculiarities of experience gained in a cultural context that strongly communicates expectations about what behaviors are morally acceptable and what not, solely on the basis of habits, traditions, rituals and conventions never critically justified.

The first two categories of the "natural"—the scientific and the statistical—are descriptive and without direct implication as to what our attitudes ought to be toward what is, according to them, either natural or unnatural. The next two—the anthropological and the conventional—are not so value-free. Already here we find judgments implied about what is "good," supposing that human interference is bad, or that which is most conventional is good. In the last two categories, we shall find these normative dimensions in the use of "natural" and "unnatural" even more prevalent and confusing.

5. *Theological.* The religious use of "natural" contrasts what is understood to be natural with the "supernatural." The natural is what occurs according to scientific natural law; the supernatural is the realm in which Divine Will works. However, these are not entirely separable, as Divine Will both creates the natural order and is capable of intervening in it, allowing exceptions or re-ordering it. The major difference between the narrowly scientific view of nature and the religious view, I suppose, is that in the scientific view, nature is seen as somehow self-ordering, through a kind of evolutionary process, whereas in what I have called the theological view, a major metaphysical leap is made when it is held that nature is ordered, re-ordered, and suspended by the working of a divine will.

An illustration here might be apt. According to the myth of creation in Genesis, God originally created the natural order such that human beings did not die. Thus human death would be *unnatural* in the scientific sense that it would not even be possible. However, after Adam and Eve's disobedience and expulsion from the Garden of Eden, God re-ordered nature so that it then became *natural* for human beings to die and *unnatural* not to do so. Sometimes, however, God makes exceptions to his natural order, temporarily suspending it, as when He takes a prophet bodily into His Kingdom (without the intervention of death) or allows Jesus to raise Lazarus from the dead. These miracles contravene, but do not alter as original sin altered, the natural order of the universe.

There is more, and what more there is makes this theology very interesting. For what comes next is the premise that *what God wills is definitive of goodness.* Scientific law, in this view, is not simply descriptive of natural reality. It is, all importantly, *regulative* of nature. Consequently, what is lawful in nature is what ought to be the case, precisely because God has willed things to be that way and what God wills defines what is good.

As near as I can make out, this is the core of reasoning at the heart of the tradition of "Natural Moral Law." Whatever else it is, "Natural Moral Law" is a theology that draws together scientific, religious, and normative premises to derive moral conclusions. Its logic is relatively clear; whether this combination of considerations ultimately makes sense is much disputed.

Some illustration of how the theological use of "natural" is used in moral reasoning might make it clearer. It seems to be especially made use of in matters of sexual morality, so let us consider what some regard as a significant moral issue, the use of contraceptives to prevent conception. On what grounds could one consider the use of either chemical or barrier (or surgical?) methods to prevent the conception of children in a world often regarded as "over-populated" to be morally wrong? One possible objection, emanating from Roman Catholic theologies, is that such techniques are "unnatural." They cannot (anymore) be regarded as "unnatural" in the sense of being either unconventional or statistically aberrant; in the anthropological sense they might be, because they are humanly induced and "artificial" means of preventing conception during intercourse. But none of these senses of "unnatural," even if they apply, yield the moral conclusion that there is something wrong with the techniques.

Rather, it is a self-consciously theological understanding of scientific naturalness that must underlie objections to contraception. More specifically, it must be some notion of what God intends that sexual capacities and sexual organs be used for that lies behind such judgments. The view is that God creates us with sexual organs for the purpose of reproducing; any other use of sexual organs violates God's desire for how they should be used and is therefore "unnatural," and therefore morally wrong. Similarly, anything that *interferes* with the proper, divinely intended use of sexual organs, as contraception surely does, will be "unnatural" and "immoral." On this basis as well it is easy to see how other (widespread) sexual practices could be regarded as immoral, for example, masturbation, oral sex, homosexuality, etc.: all involve a use of sexual organs for purposes other than that purpose for which God intended they be used, in ways in which conception cannot occur, and are thus "unnatural" (even "perversions") and morally wrong.[7]

Similarly, suicide is sometimes regarded as wrong because it is "unnatural," and "unnatural" in that it is contrary to a "will to live" that each person is supposed to have "naturally." And again, the only sense of "natural" that will work here to yield the desired moral judgment is one in which it is supposed that God creates us with a "natural will to live" because it his intention that we do so to serve some purpose of His. To act contrary to this desire of God's, by willfully seeking to end one's own life, is "unnatural" and therefore morally wrong.[8]

6. *Evaluative* (Moral). Far the most difficult category of use for "natural" is the straightforwardly evaluative. This may be because there is no

simple use of "natural" that is readily equatable with a judgment of value. Most such judgments, at least, are arrived at by collapsing together two different categories, for example, the conventional and the moral. Thus what is conventionally "natural" will be taken to be, without further consideration or argument, morally correct. ("We have always done things this way"—held slaves, practiced clitorectomy, bound feet, etc. "It is the natural and correct way for things to be.") Or what usually happens, statistically, will be supposed to be regulative of how things ought to be. ("Historically, nearly all societies have been class-stratified. This is a natural and morally justifiable social order.") Or some general bias against human interference in the "natural order" will lead one to suppose all such actions "unnatural" and bad. ("If God had meant there to be more light during the day, He would have made days longer. Daylight savings time is unnatural and wrong.") But in such cases, as Veatch observes, "one conception of the natural provides the content for another," and this can only lead to confusion.[9]

Again, numerous things fall simultaneously into two or more categories, and this may cause confusion when the "natural" and the "moral" are equated. An example of multiple categorization is "Air is naturally (biologically, statistically) colorless." This sort of dual categorization causes no problems. Problems do arise, however, when one of the categories is moral, as in "Child molestation is unnatural (statistically, conventionally, morally)." The danger is then that a moral judgment needing (and capable of) rational justification will simply be assumed, because "unnatural" in some other sense than "moral" will be allowed to carry the weight.

If this were all there were to a moral sense of "unnatural," then its use would always be either confused or question-begging. But morality is sufficiently complex, and moral theory more than sufficiently difficult, that one should not be sanguine in placing too great an emphasis upon the need for (and possibility of) rationally justifying every value judgment. Great reliance is still frequently placed upon "self-evident truths" and "intuitions" in moral reasoning. And where such language as this is at home, there is "naturally" (conventionally) room as well for "natural" and "unnatural" as moral categories. For in this context, "natural" is a synonym for "self-evident" or "intuitively known," and if these latter two terms are admissible in moral discourse, so too is "natural."

Be this as it may, the limitations of "natural" and "unnatural" as moral predicates are severe, and their use far more frequently obscures than illuminates matters. This being so, we would be far further ahead abjuring their use wherever possible. This is no less true for their use in discussions of death than it is in the discourse of morality. And where evaluations of modes of dying or the status of death itself are at issue, there is double reason to avoid the use of "natural" and "unnatural" altogether.

But unfortunately, again, this is not all there is to the matter. To leave it at this point, with the understanding that the use of "natural" as a moral predicate is confused or question-begging and always obfuscating would not be fair to its highly sophisticated theological uses. So before fully abandoning "natural" and its cognates as a useful notion, it would be well to consider further its theological uses.

Theological Uses of
"Natural" Reconsidered

Earlier I characterized the theological use of "natural" as a blend of scientific, moral, and religious understandings. To see more adequately how these work together it is necessary, still again, to look at the argument that seeks to show death is not an evil because it is a natural biological reality. A deeper probing of that argument will show its essential theological foundations, and will enable us better to evaluate these. It will also allow us to go beyond the superficial criticisms of that position offered in chapter one. There I objected that the view that death was to be "accepted," resting on an argument such as this one, had some very undesirable moral and political implications, that it gave encouragement to repressive and oppressive forces in the status quo. Furthermore, I thought that in urging passive acceptance of death it forced still greater hardship upon those who had suffered most the injustices of the status quo. True as I believe all that to be, it must be acknowledged that showing a view to be dangerous is something less than showing it to be false. The present examination, I hope, will come closer to doing the latter.[10]

What we are considering is the drawing of an inference that death is not an evil and should be accepted from the claim that death is a natural biological fact. The full statement of such a view requires filling in 2 below as a suppressed premise:

1. Death is a natural biological fact, necessary, inevitable, and inescapable for all living organisms.

2. Whatever is necessary, inevitable, and inescapable is good, or at least not evil, and should be accepted.

3. Therefore, death must be seen as either good, or at least not evil, and must be accepted.

The fallacy in this argument is readily seen if one substitutes for death some other "natural fact." According to one's biases, any of the following are plausible candidates: the extinguishing of the sun and destruction of the earth, war, murder, suicide, homosexuality, oncogenes, genetic disease, and so on. If one is determined to keep the domain to strictly *biological* natural facts, the last two in our list will suffice. In any case, however "natural" these may be, it is clear this is no warrant for regarding them as "good" and "acceptable."

Leon Kass has defended a version of the argument above, and his reply to this objection is that the sorts of substitutions suggested here for "death" are not natural in the way death is natural, for they are none of them "as natural, necessary and inextricably bound up with life as [is] death . . . ." All these have "natural causes," but they are not "encoded in the genome that 'contains the information' for the other processes of life."

> [W]hereas both disease and decline have "natural" causes, much disease is caused at least in part by external agency, and the body responds to disease by "attempting" to heal itself, to make itself healthy, to make itself whole. In this sense, disease is *fought* by nature working within, whereas decline is *produced* by nature working within. . . . unlike all those other things which occur in life, decline and death are part of life, an integral part which cannot be extruded without destroying the whole.[11]

It is tempting to regard this as simply obscurantism, as mystifying and possibly mystical layerings of "natural." For after all, genetic anomalies (present in every human being) and genetic diseases (those genetic anomalies that work especially severe hardship on their carriers) are "encoded in the genome" and "produced by nature working within." This is no reason to suppose them "good." Oncogenes at the very least provide one with an increased susceptibility to developing cancer, and deficiencies in one's immunological responses to potent viruses can be devastating. Recently, even aging—surely a paradigm of higher order "naturalness" in Kass's ontology—has been argued to be more like than unlike disease, and a potentially "curable condition."[12]

But I do not think it simple obscurantism at work behind such views as these. Rather, I think there is a hidden premise, one both theological and normative, that undergirds premise 2 in the argument above. It is the premise that allows for equating the "natural" and the "good." The suppressed notion is that whatever happens consonant with the deepest and most general principles of natural order is good because these principles are not themselves accidental or fortuitous. Rather, principles of natural order are created by a benign (read: divine) being as expressions of His will, and as such are definitive of goodness. From this it of course follows that whatever is natural, in the sense of being the embodiment of a good God's will, is good.

This view does make possible the equating of the "natural" with the "good" and allows the argument for the naturalness and acceptability of death to proceed. But what might be problematical about this theological underpinning itself? At least two serious difficulties can be alleged that will need to be addressed by its defenders.

The first difficulty to be addressed is the rather peculiar view of "natural (scientific) law" this theology embodies. It seems to conflate scientific law with moral law as equally expressions of divine will. They may both be regarded as expressions of divine will, but this will not by itself allow that they be essentially identical. Scientific law, at least as understood by science, is not regulative or prescriptive; it does not determine how natural events "ought to" or "must" occur. Scientific law is rather our best understanding of how nature works in fact; it is a description of what occurs and not a prescription of how it ought to or must occur. As such, it presupposes no need for a "law-giver," as all regulative law—whether customary, civil, or moral—does.

A direct implication of this scientific as distinct from theological understanding of natural law is that evaluative judgments about whether it is a good or a bad thing are entirely inappropriate, are, if one likes, "category mistakes," rather like attributing colors to concepts. In attempting to articulate an understanding of how nature works, scientists are of course guided by values in their selection of data and in their formulation of what problems are worth pursuing. So I am not claiming science to be "value-free," "neutral," or altogether "objective." But in putting forth those understandings of nature, formulated as natural laws, there is no notion that these laws are guidelines for how nature ought to act, in the way rules of etiquette, the criminal law, and principles of morality are imperatives for human behavior.

The second difficulty is an ancient one, with us at least since Socrates. In *Euthyphro,* Socrates explores with a pious young man the nature of "Goodness." Euthyphro is quite certain he knows what it is, even after Socrates leads him through numerous dialectical traps. Euthyphro's best formulation is that what is good is what God loves, desires, or, as we might put it, commands. This leads Socrates to formulate a dilemma, as pertinent today for what are called "divine command theories of morality" as it was 2500 years ago. Let us grant that whatever God commands is good, and that whatever is good God commands. But in which direction, as it were, does the causal arrow point? Does God command that which is good because it is good, or is it good because God commands it? If the former, it is not God's willing something to be the case that makes that thing good, and we might discover what it is about a thing that makes it good independently of God's willing it. But if the latter, then it is God's willing something to be so that makes it a good state of affairs. However, the difficulty now is that what is "good" may be entirely arbitrary.

If one is not bothered by the possibility of all moral principles being arbitrary and potentially whimsical, it would be worth reflecting on what a fragile enterprise morality is to begin with. Our best insights into standards of decency and behavior respectful of the personhood of others have been hard won and never very secure in a world ruled more by power than by moral principle. A theology that further endangers and undermines our efforts to create moral standards by finally characterizing them as entirely arbitrary expressions of divine will (perhaps even of raw power) does not serve us well. Among other things, it is singularly insensitive to the real moral dilemma Abraham found himself in when, first among God's chosen people, God commanded Abraham to kill Isaac on the sacrificial altar.[13]

I raise these issues of the understanding of natural law and of the relation of divine will to goodness not as refutations of the view that the scientifically natural is necessarily good, but as difficulties that any such theology must grapple with. For those determined to see a "natural harmony" in the universe which integrates science and morality and emanates from divine creation, these are very serious problems. The rest of us, rapidly approaching the twenty-first century and finding such a world view unpersuasive, must seek other ways of understanding the relation between nature and goodness. My own preference, in light of the ambiguity and confusion that surrounds "natural," is to abandon it as an evaluative term, especially as a moral predicate. This will not be altogether possible, however, until we consider further its uses with "death" and "dying," specifically, with "good death" and "good dying."

Natural Death, Dying Naturally, and Good Death

In light of the foregoing analysis, how should we now understand such a claim as "A natural death is a good death"? In the first place, it would be well to be clear whether someone saying this is really talking about death as such, or rather the process leading up to death known as dying. Aside from the confusion engendered by collapsing "natural" and "good" together, there is the further difficulty of ascertaining whether it is really death one is speaking of or dying. When claiming a natural death is a good death, sometimes people really do mean that death is good, perhaps because it came at the end of a dying that was so terrible. But sometimes also one might use "good death" as shorthand for a dying process judged to be good (or easy, or peaceful, or dignified, or natural, etc.) for the person now dead or for survivors.

I have said all I think needs saying about the supposition that death as such is good in any circumstances: it is not, even though it may not be the worst thing that happens to one. But this will not settle in the least the questions of how dying can be good or ill, whether dying naturally is good, and what "dying naturally" might mean. It is to these questions that we must now turn. Necessarily, we must begin with the last of these questions first: What does "natural dying" or "dying naturally" mean?

It would be banal and boring to insist that dying is scientifically natural; it could not be otherwise. By "natural dying" must be meant either how most people die (statistical), or a dying that is familiar to us (conventional), or dying that is not artificially prolonged by humanly manipulated technologies (anthropological). Any or all of these could then be taken as equivalent to "good dying" in an evaluative sense (moral).

Why we should want to do this, however, is somewhat more difficult to fathom. Why it might be assumed, for instance, that dying as most people die is a good thing is especially problematical. For most people may well die before they want to, or before their sense of completing life has been achieved, or in agonizing pain or despair, or insensible to their condition, as burdens to their survivors or leaving others in deep despair, and so on.

Rather more plausible candidates for equating "natural dying" with "good dying" are those deaths that do not shock our socially conditioned sensibilities and those that are not drawn out pointlessly and painfully by the use of life-prolonging (or rather, death-delaying) technologies. These may well be important considerations in the evaluation of dying as good or bad. I think they are. But the issue right here is not whether these are relevant features of any dying that might justifiably be called a good dying, but whether they are properly identified as relevant features of a good death (i.e., dying) by calling them "natural dying" or "natural death." For three reasons, I believe they are not.

In the first place, it is undesirable to use "natural death" as an evaluative phrase, precisely because of the multiplicity of meanings of "natural," several of which are far removed from any evaluative sense. Considerable confusion and lack of clarity can result from such a mix.

In the second place, using "natural" as an evaluative term, as already demonstrated, grievously begs the question as to whether a thing is good or bad. There may be some occasions when it is legitimate to regard a value judgment as correct because "self-evident" or "intuitively known"; and it may accordingly be legitimate to use "natural" as a synonym for "self-evident" and "intuitively known." But there are not many such occasions, and fewer still in which "natural" is used in this manner. For the most part, "natural" in one sense, for example, the conventional, is taken to provide the content for "natural" in an evaluative sense. This begs the question precisely because there is no warrant for generally supposing that because something is familiar to us it is good. Much more must go into a justified judgment of value than this.

Finally, even in those uses of "natural death" which are closest to being evaluative—the conventional and the anthropological—there is such extraordinary variety of meaning and subjectivity that they are unsuitable candidates for bringing light to the difficult notion of "good dying." Consider, for example, this account of "natural death" by George Orwell, relating his experience in a French hospital in 1929:

> I had seen dead men before . . . usually men who had died violent deaths. Numero 57's eyes were still open, his mouth also open, his small face contorted into an expression of agony. What most impressed me, however, was the whiteness of his face. It had been pale before, but now it was little darker than the sheets. As I gazed at the tiny, screwed-up face it struck me that this disgusting piece of refuse, waiting to be carted

away and dumped on a slab in the dissecting room, was an example of "natural" death, one of the things you pray for in the Litany. There you are then, I thought, that's what is waiting for you, twenty, thirty, forty years hence: that is how the lucky ones die, the one who lives to be old. . . . People talk about the horrors of war, but what weapon has man invented that even approaches in cruelty some of the commoner diseases? "Natural" death, almost by definition, means something low, smelly, and painful.[14]

The variability of customs and the subjectivity of what is counted as not humanly interfered with I have supposed make both conventional and anthropological senses of "natural" unsuitable for regarding "natural death" or "natural dying" in either of these senses desirable candidates for evaluating "good death" or "good dying." There are those, however, who might take this variability and subjectivity as *advantages* just because it would show the impossibility of objectively generalizing about what might count as good dying. I think this a serious issue, but am not yet prepared to yield to such a perspective. Until we have considered separately and carefully the notion of "good dying," as we shall attempt to do in the next chapter, it would be premature to suppose that no rational evaluation is even possible, and that all we can hope for is an endless variety of subjective judgments.

What must finally be clear, however, if this analysis and these arguments show anything, is that notions of "natural death" and "natural dying," whether or not equated with "good death" or "good dying," are very unsuitable for doing any of the five tasks earlier listed as being among those such language has been used to do: asserting a right, illuminating an ideal, formulating guidelines for when to initiate or discontinue life-prolonging treatments in medicine, shaping public policy, or serving in coherent arguments for how to regard death.

As an illustration of this conclusion, consider only the uses of "natural death" in medicine, where it is frequently invoked as an aid in deciding whether it is worthwhile to use "artificial" means to prolong life, possibly at the expense of a terminally ill person's "dignity." Put in this manner, few would doubt that "natural death" (anthropologically, evaluatively) would be desirable, and hence medicine ought to back off and "let nature take its course." But what of the kind of "natural death" Orwell describes, which is surely no less horrific than the vision provoked above of a dying person filled with needles and tubes, fluids flowing in and out, ventilators pumping away, monitors buzzing, whirring, humming, and clicking, and so on? One of the things all of us want medicine to do is to intervene to modify the sort of "natural dying" Orwell describes, to mitigate the suffering and indignity of such a demise. But equally, one of the other things we frequently want medicine to do is not to intervene aggressively and futilely to prolong a "natural dying" that cannot be other than postponed at great expense to the comfort and dignity of a terminally ill person. What is made clear by such desires, or better, moral convictions, is that a notion of "natural dying," by itself, cannot guide us in determining what ought to be done. On the contrary, it only obscures the real issues, making thoughtful decision making more difficult. Hence we would be better off abandoning talk of what is "natural" or "unnatural" in dying in favor of directly considering what would count as "good dying."

VI

GOOD DYING

The busy day, the peaceful night,
Unfelt, uncounted glided by;
His frame was firm, his powers were bright
Tho' now his eightieth year was nigh.
Then with no throbbing fiery pain,
No cold gradations of decay,
Death broke at once the vital chain,
And free'd his soul the nearest way.

Samuel Johnson
On the Death of Dr. Robert Levet

. . . and spare us, Oh Lord, from the evil
of sudden death.
Rogation Day Prayer

If death is not good, dying might still be so. "Good death" makes most sense when it is elliptical speech for "good dying," when not the achievement or event of death is judged to be good, but rather the process of arriving there is what is being evaluated. In the previous chapter, two conclusions stand out: first, that "good dying" is not illuminated by equating it with "natural death"; and second, that it is vitally important to be clear about what is meant by and counts as good dying in understanding important assertions of rights (a right to die), ideals (dying well, or as one ought), and guides for public policy and for making treatment decisions in medicine (pronouncing death, disconnecting ventilators, whether to initiate chemotherapy, stopping efforts at providing nutrition and hydration, etc.). Accordingly, we shall seek again to understand the concept of good dying.

Judgments about good dying, however, are as diverse and problem-laden as are notions of natural death. In the first place, at least three obvious things might be meant by "good dying": that a particular dying process was good for the person who experienced it directly, that it was good for those who experienced it indirectly and survived, or that it was in accord with some standard of social probity and the dying person could be said to have done it well. Beyond this, there are very diverse notions of goodness at work when evaluating dying. For the time being at least, we shall be concerned with analyzing and evaluating notions of good dying that address all three of these sets of interests.

There seem at the present moment to be three paradigms for a person's dying experience to be regarded as a good one, in the sense of an ideal we might aspire to achieve or otherwise be fortunate to experience. The candidates for good dying are (1) sudden death, (2) "appropriate" death, and (3) death with dignity. Each of these will require analysis and evaluation, for each has been strongly advocated.

Sudden Death

Most people die, but not all. Some are killed, or become dead very quickly, in which case they experience little or no dying. One moment a person is alive, the next he is dead, as in the poet's account of Dr. Levet's death. And on some accounts this is certainly the best way to become dead—suddenly, and, if one is fortunate, peacefully and painlessly, perhaps quietly slipping away, unaware of what is happening, while asleep, with no preceding and prolonged period of decline. A sudden death that is quiet and easy might be equated with euthanasia, in its original meaning. Euthanasia, from the Greek eu (good) and thanatos (death), is taken to mean simply a quiet and easy death, shorn of all controversial complications of the moral permissibility of anyone helping another to achieve this good dying. The obvious appeal of this mode of death as an ideal of good dying is that one who dies suddenly is spared the often considerable trauma of increasing decline and disability, of prolonged pain and psychological terror, of difficult partings with those who will live on, even of responsibility for consciously finishing up one's life. Slipping out the back door of a party, or life itself, can avoid many difficulties of leave-taking.

Many people in the United States, if pressed on how they would prefer to die if they must do so in the very near future, say "suddenly." Besides the desire to avoid suffering on their part, they give as an additional reason for such a preference their belief that such a death would be easier for their family and friends to deal with: they too would be spared the agony of enduring a long dying for someone they love. Thus for both self-centered and other-regarding reasons, sudden death is frequently advanced as a model of good dying.

To give sudden death its strongest formulation as an ideal, it is perhaps necessary to add a few other qualifiers. One might stipulate that it occur only when one is very old and has accomplished one's life's work; after one's moral obligations to others for whom one has responsibility have been discharged; in circumstances where one's death will not shock or outrage survivors, and so on. In short, all the conditions that Callahan stipulates as desirable for a "natural death" might be attached to sudden death to entice us to believe it is the ideal dying.[1]

But this is something of a cheat. These additional features are of the sort that could be readily added to any proposed ideal of good dying, and are in no way unique to sudden death. If we are to understand and evaluate sudden death—or for that matter, appropriate death or death with dignity—as an ideal dying, we must focus upon the characteristics unique to that model and set aside those shared with virtually all others. In the end, we will, of course, have to consider what features, if any, are universalizable to a reasonable ideal of good dying.

Are the reasons for preferring sudden death to all other forms of dying compelling? I do not think so, for three reasons. In the first place, one might feel, with supplicants of old, that, all things considered, it would be better to be spared "the evil of sudden death." Dying is sometimes called "the final phase of life," and while it is almost certainly not the most pleasant phase, it may still be among the most important. For it is in that final phase that many people find the opportunity to assess their lives for meaningfulness; bring closure to activities, strivings and relationships; make arrangements so their deaths will not unduly inconvenience, discomfort, or distress those they love; seek reconciliation with friends, enemies, and God. To be deprived of the opportunity to do these sorts of things, because one dies unaware of what is happening, is a very great loss.

The loss is not one's own alone. Those who live on suffer too, and frequently suffer a great deal more for another's death having come so suddenly that they could not anticipate or prepare for it. We know enough now about the phenomenology of grieving to know that grief is more endurable for those who have the opportunity to anticipate loss and psychologically prepare for bereavement.[2] Other-regarding considerations argue against, not for, sudden death.

Finally, there is a perhaps somewhat eccentric consideration, having to do with awareness and consciousness itself. For nonhedonists, who prefer Socrates' injunction to live the examined life and to "know thyself" as opposed to avoiding unpleasantness at all cost, awareness of even unpleasant changes in life heralding death is a positive value. To slip away, in one's sleep, unawares—all desirable features of a dying that is sudden—are themselves a kind of evil, the evil of not knowing what is happening to one's very own self. Having such knowledge is almost certainly not enjoyable, but it is vitally important. Not to have awareness of anything so central to one's being as the end of that being would be a terrible thing. On this account, it is not that awareness of impending death has any practical value for oneself or others, but rather that such awareness is *intrinsically* valuable to a self-conscious human being.

In conclusion, it might be supposed that sudden death is attractive only from within a mystique (or even a fully developed culture) of death denial. Such a mystique is itself not a good thing, for, as suggested in chapter one, it sustains the illusion that death is unreal and only ever accidental, and it badly prepares us for coping with the harsher realities of living, including, most especially, the reality of the dying each of us is most likely to experience. Suffering, while never unreservedly a good thing or good in itself, is often a means to good ends in the far from perfect world we live in. And the suffering inescapable in dying, as opposed to its avoidance through becoming dead all at once, is a suffering with potentially enormous benefits, some few of which were considered above.

Appropriate Death

"Appropriate death" is a term coined by Avery Weisman and used by him to specify "a death that someone might choose for himself—had he a choice."[3] If this were all Weisman meant by appropriate death, one might think that he intended its use, instead of "good death" or "good dying," as a way of avoiding the laying on of moral requirements for dying well. This impression is reinforced by Weisman's very outspoken assertion that "To tell another person what he ought to do, think, or be is an affront at any time; but to do this when he nears the end of life is sanctimonious cruelty" (p. 36).

So understood, appropriate death appears to be a respectful way of deferring to a dying person's own judgment of what would be, for her or for him, a good way of dying. Different people, with very diverse experiences, relationships, attitudes, and values, will surely regard their dying differently. Some might prefer sudden death, because, say, they have always lived life actively avoiding unpleasantness and psychologically denying difficulties. Others, deeply rooted in a set of familial relationships, might want most that their dying be easy on those they love, and are little concerned with their own comfort or longevity. Still others might care most about the salvation of their souls, and would want to know what is happening to them that they might repent and be saved. There is no one set of requirements possible for a good dying, and the best we can do is hope that everyone attain an appropriate death, one consistent with their individual values and choices.

There is certainly much to be said for avoiding "sanctimonius cruelty" and for respecting an individual's own evaluation of what is required for his or her dying to be as good a one as possible. It is not clear, however, that Weisman's notion of appropriate death will do either of these things. On the one hand, it is not itself free of normative, prescriptive judgments about what counts as good dying, and on the other hand, no notion of good dying could or even should try to be free of some such judgments in favor of the rampant relativism that allows whatever anyone chooses to be sufficient for calling it "good." Insofar as Weisman's explanation of appropriate death is itself fraught with prescriptions of how the dying ought to behave, he violates his own requirements; and insofar as it lacks some standards of value, it would not be useful.

In an article published soon after *On Dying and Denying*, Weisman characterizes appropriate death as follows:

> Appropriate deaths are those in which suffering is at a low ebb, conflict is minimal, and behavior has been maintained on as high a level as is compatible with physical status. Moreover, the dying patient indicates that what has already been done corresponds to what he expected of himself, of the people who matter most, of those to whom he turned for relief, and finally, of the world in general. Literally and metaphorically, it is time to die. Relief of anguish and resolution of remaining conflicts join in a harmonious exitus. The patient both accepts and expects death, and is willing, albeit ruefully, to die. It is the ultimate of successful coping. [4]

And in *On Dying and Denying* itself, Weisman undertakes to advise caretakers for the terminally ill on their duties:

> Someone who dies an appropriate death must be helped in the following ways: He should be relatively pain-free, his suffering reduced, and emotional and social impoverishments kept to a minimum. Within the limits of disability, he should operate on as high and effective a level as possible, even though only tokens of former fulfillments can be offered. He should also recognize and resolve residual conflicts, and satisfy whatever remaining wishes are consistent with his present plight and with his ego ideal. Finally, among his choices, he should be able to yield control to others in whom he has confidence. He also has the option of asking or relinquishing significant key people. [5]

The plethora of value judgments and prescriptions about how dying persons ought best behave in the above hardly needs enumeration. It is worth observing, however, that the initial impression that "appropriate death" was intended as a mechanism to avoid laying on the dying the expectations of others of how they ought best behave and to respect their individuality is mistaken. For here Weisman is quite clear in his articulation of values concerning professional caretakers, their duties, the obligations of "patients" to be conforming, the desirability of ascribing to a mystique of accepting death, and so on. Weisman seems initially to recognize the problematical nature of prescribing moral requirements for dying for those with diminishing power to do anything, least of all fulfill the stringent requirements of morality. Yet this does not prevent him from putting forth such requirements, and in a particularly demanding way at that.

But if Weisman's explication of a notion of "appropriate death" violates his own injunction not to impose upon the dying the expectations of others on how they ought to die, it does not follow that the notion is necessarily invalidated. As a purely sociological observation, it has merit: people do indeed, in the ordinary course of events, die as they live. If one has been greedy in living, one is likely to be greedy in dying; if generous throughout life, generous in dying. As a part of life, dying is to a very significant degree consonant with living. And while few can choose the precise means or time of death, all can, to some greater or lesser extent, choose how to respond to fate. In this sense, however one chooses to confront death, as long as it is consistent with one's living, will be an appropriate death.

But it is not sociological observation alone or even chiefly that a notion of appropriate death is intended to serve. Rather, it is supposed to offer us some vision of what would be a desirable mode of dying, insofar as dying can be done well or experienced with the least possible distress. In that respect, the notion of appropriate death seems simply to assert that the best dying is the dying each of us would choose for her or himself, if we could choose, and no other considerations are relevant. As such, it places not merely paramount, but exclusive, emphasis upon the importance of self-determination and autonomy in determining what for each person will count as a good dying. Is this sufficient?

It is worth remembering that a notion of good dying must serve three constituencies: the interests of the dying person, the interests of those who love that person, and the interests of a larger community, expressed as moral expectations of how one ought to behave while dying. This revised concept of appropriate death now under consideration is profoundly skeptical of these last interests, altogether indifferent to the second, and exclusively centered on the first, the interests of the dying person. How should we regard this approach?

This revised version of appropriate death has significant strengths. Chief among them is its perception of the centrality of respecting self-determining choices in defining the interest of another, even, or perhaps especially, the interests of one who is dying. Such respect for autonomy is central to the moral requirement of respecting the personhood of another. Moreover, its skepticism about the propriety, even the justness, of setting forth moral requirements for good dying is by and large a healthy one. Dying is a progressive loss of power and renders one ever less able to handle "obligations," including obligations on how best to die. Such decline and diminishment requires deference, not the imposition of ever more difficult moral duties.

But even this revised version of appropriate death has significant weaknesses as well. The most glaring of these is its seeming indifference to the interests of those who will live on after someone they love has died. Such persons are deeply involved in a dying that, while not wholly their own, takes from them something of immense value. This degree of loss is itself a kind of dying, and it too demands consideration.

No dying that leaves survivors unconsolably distraught, outraged, or bitter can really be regarded as a good one, however much it may have been desired, chosen, even brought about by the deceased. In some cases, suicide is the ultimate expression of self-determination in death. If self-determination were all that was required for good dying, suicide would be our paradigm. Whatever else we may think of suicide, we cannot often suppose it good for those left behind, and we cannot possibly be comfortable with indifference to their needs and interests.

This suggests a further deficiency in the revised view of appropriate death. Not merely does it suffer from undue disregard for the interests of others, but it seems as well not to have a very well developed conception of the dying person's interests. Precisely because to die is to experience ever diminishing powers of agency, self-determination for the dying is not always desired, possible, or even in the dying person's interest. Sometimes being sensitively cared for, having decisions made by others, experiencing others doing for one what one can no longer do for oneself—all these are better than autonomous self-determination.

In sum, this revised concept of appropriate death, as a model for good dying suffers the ills of all ethical positions predicated exclusively on emphasizing autonomy: it shows too little regard for others, has too narrow a view of the dying person's interests, and invites a far too sweeping moral skepticism about what standards of behavior and moral value can be reasonably endorsed. But it does get us closer to a reasonable perspective on good dying, even if only by distorting considerations that put in the proper perspective are crucially important. Among these are its insistence on respecting the self-determined choices of one who is dying, and its reluctance to endorse unattainable standards of behavior for such persons. Perhaps in the concept of death with dignity we will find a point of view on good dying that builds on the strengths of notions of sudden death and appropriate death but avoids their pitfalls.

Death with Dignity

Notions of sudden death and appropriate death as models of good dying are relatively simple and straightforward; death with dignity is a far more complex, even convoluted, concept. Clearly this difficulty has to do with different uses, and therefore different meanings, of "dignity." The situation, however, is not nearly as unmanageable as understanding the uses, misuses, and conflicts that arise with "natural." This is because, I believe, the relevant uses of "dignity" are related in ways that uses of "natural" are not, so that it is quite possible to salvage from these various uses of "dignity" some clear applications to concerns with rights, ideals, and grounds for moral and political evaluation with which we began.

Unlike the uses of "natural," the various uses of "dignity" as it is used in connection with "death" bear a discernible connection to its root meaning. The Latin word *dignitas* denotes honorableness, worth, excellence, and desert; it applies to persons of high rank or estate (dignitaries). Such persons are expected to have a nobility of manner or style. In our more democratic age, however, "dignity" has been spread about (some no doubt would say diluted), so that in certain crucial respects it is held to belong to every person. The most vital dimensions of dignity, especially in "dying with dignity" or "death with dignity," seem to be the following:[6]

1. *Consciousness and Rationality*. It is often supposed, following Aristotle, that the distinctive "dignity" of humankind is precisely its consciousness, especially consciousness of self, and its capacity for rationality. Rationality not only distinguishes us from all other species, its exercise is our most noble achievement. Consciousness and the capacity for rationality constitute human dignity in the most generic sense, for all those we would be prepared to call persons. Without consciousness and, to a lesser degree, the capacity for rationality, we do not have personhood.

It is this dimension of human dignity that underlies contemporary efforts to redefine fundamentally the criteria for determining death. Notions of "brain death" and the use of such notions for declaring death have less to do with when "in fact" death occurs than they do with an evaluative judgment of when distinctively human life and all possiblity of dignified human life have been lost. It is thought an *indignity*, a moral offense, disrespectful of the person who was, to further sustain such biological processes as respiration and heartbeat when all consciousness is permanently gone. "Death with dignity" in such cases means discontinuing the insult of sustaining the biological processes of a person who no longer exists. The dead deserve the respect of being disposed of in a proper manner, and of not being pointlessly maintained or, worse yet, exploited for the benefit of others.[7]

2. *Self-determination* (Autonomy). Next to consciousness itself, surely the most important dimension of human dignity is self-determination. The opportunity to make one's own choices and to implement these without interference by others is a freedom that human beings have long struggled to attain. Its deprivation can be devastating to those who have known it, and in the name of preserving or attaining it many, ironically, have died. According the power of self-determination to persons is an enormous enhancement to dignity, so much so that it is sometimes taken to be definitive of human dignity. Those who have suffered imprisonment, slavery, or other deprivations of liberty have often been keenly aware of how serious a threat to their dignity such oppression is.

3. *Bodily Integrity*. Well enculturated human beings typically place enormous value upon how they physically appear to others. Vast resources are invested in the decorative arts of makeup, clothing, hair styling, jewelry, and so on. Similarly, control of one's bodily movements and processes is thought central to one's self-esteem, sense of worth, and dignity. Disease itself, and dying even more than disease, are assaults upon bodily integrity, and thereby are inherently undignified. Disease all too often disfigures and debilitates; dying always does so. Both radically

alter appearance and diminish control over movement, through impaired neurological systems or weakened muscles. Disease and dying can make bodily processes, such as respiration, dependent upon drugs or machines, and can destroy bladder and bowel control. They almost invariably lessen our attractiveness to others and to ourselves. These are all serious assaults upon bodily integrity, and therefore as well upon human dignity.

4. *Self-esteem*. How one feels about one's self is an important aspect of human dignity. It very greatly influences how one behaves, whether with a sense of worth or not, whether with pride or not. Self-esteem is closely connected with dignity, in the root sense of "nobility," in which demeanor is crucial. One's sense of worthiness and self-respect is not, for the most part, internally generated; it very greatly depends upon how one is regarded in the larger community. Social position and reputation, therefore, influence dignity, almost to the point that we might say that to this extent dignity is conferred upon one by the social order. Yet to experience this dimension of dignity is very much a subjective sense of who one is.

Bodily integrity is an important aspect of human dignity, both because it is so widely valued by human beings and because it is vital to our very existence. But it should be noted that it, like self-esteem, is a far more subjective ground for dignity than the generic foundation of consciousness and rationality. The relationship of bodily integrity to self-esteem is highly variable, as people regard their bodies in very divergent ways. I met a man in Houston, for instance, who acquired a pair of new shoes that were far too small for him. They were very difficult to get back on once removed, so he did not take them off. Soon after acquiring the shoes, he went on an alcoholic binge. Ten days later he could not stand up, as his feet were too swollen and painful, so he was taken to a Veteran's Administration hospital. There the shoes had to be cut off. The doctors found his feet to be badly infected and infested with maggots. Many observers were appalled by his condition; he was not. This elderly gentleman was unfazed by the condition of his feet or the causes. Despite all explanations to the contrary, he insisted his injuries must have occurred when a car ran over his feet. Nothing could penetrate this defense, and he continued to conduct himself with the utmost sense of pride, of dignity, even of grandeur befitting his status as a veteran of foreign wars!

On the other hand, I have known any number of young people who quite seriously claim that they would rather die than suffer the humiliation of any, even relatively minor, bodily impairment, such as the loss of all their hair. Now it may well be that the gentleman above is self-deceived, and those who would prefer death to disfigurement naive or suffering under a strange system of values. But in each case, their own subjective sense of what is central to their dignity as persons is strong.

Again, individuals differ enormously on how important self-determination is to them. For the rampant individualist, it is all important; others are only too content to be dependent and taken care of by friends or strangers; for rational persons, self-determination is to be assessed in conjunction with other goods, such as bodily integrity and self-esteem. Consciousness and autonomy are most important, even indispensable to human dignity, but some degree of bodily integrity and self-esteem are also important. And while we may individually give different weights to each of these, and emphasize one more than others, all are requisite for the fullest conception of human dignity.

It is the emphasizing of one dimension of dignity over others that leads to very different evaluations of what is required for persons to die with dignity. There is, perhaps, least controversy now about the centrality of consciousness, so that few have any difficulty removing certifiably "brain-dead" persons from life support systems. Where consciousness is only partially impaired, as in various forms of dementia, there is far more conflict. All can agree that human dignity has been diminished for those whose consciousness is partially impaired, but we cannot agree how significant such diminishment is to decisions about how aggressively to pursue the goal of sustaining bodily integrity for such persons. And most tragically, the demented dying themselves cannot tell us how important consciousness is to them, for they are unable to make such an evaluation.

Autonomy with respect to dying has most to do not with choosing death but with the decisions one is able to make while dying. We cannot help but die, choose it or otherwise. But in dying there are numerous decisions to be made, often about how long to take in dying, whether to use death delaying therapies, how highly to prize pain control over full awareness, where to die, how much weight to give to the interests of others, even such seemingly small matters as what to eat and when. These are the sorts of decisions one either does or does not participate in making. But the more one participates in making such decisions, the more one's dignity as a self-determining human being is recognized and respected. Very often, the demand to die with dignity, phrased as a right to do so, is just this insistence that the dying are entitled to control as many of the circumstances of their own dying as they are capable and desirous of controlling.

Given this analysis of "death with dignity," can we hope to do the most important things which the discourse of death with dignity has been called upon to do? That is, can this analysis of dignified dying be used to support the assertion of a right to die with dignity, guide public policy, help in making medical treatment decisions for the terminally ill, and articulate an ideal, or at least desirable, mode of dying, and the like? My temporizing answer to this query is a qualified affirmative one: it will do some of these things, but will not be sufficient by itself to do any of them fully. Consider, in turn, a right to die with dignity, medicine and dignified dying, and dignified dying as an ideal.

The Right to Die with Dignity

Sometimes it is a putative "right to die" *simpliciter* that is asserted, and that is surely a baffling claim. In the first place, two quite different things might be meant: either that one has a right to achieve death, or that one has a right to a dying process. If it is a "right" to attain death one is asserting, the obvious question is why would anyone want to claim a "right"—moral or legal—to something they cannot possibly fail to attain? Death is in this respect asymmetrical with life: being alive is accidental, fortuitous, and, to a greater or lesser degree, always tenuous. It therefore makes considerable sense to affirm that those who are alive have a right to remain so (everything else being equal). But there is surely no such tenuousness about death, and hardly a need to assert a right to something that, wanted or not, will come our way.

On the other hand, it is hardly less puzzling to assert that one has a right to a dying process. What kind of right is this, a "liberty" right, or an "entitlement" right? That is, is the right to a dying process the sort of good one should be allowed without interference by others, or is it the sort of good that others are obligated to assure that one achieves? But who, really, would suppose that dying completely unattended to by others was desirable and a "right," and how could we possibly go about assuring everyone that death would not for them be sudden, and that they would, as a matter of right, experience dying? The "right to die" construed as a liberty right is patently undesirable, and construed as an entitlement right, impossible.

Consequently, it is not a right to die as such that is intended by such discourse. Rather, what seems to be meant is that persons have a right to die *in a certain way*, that way most frequently characterized as "with dignity." This claim, whatever its merits, at least makes sense. For now what is being affirmed is that persons have a right to exercise some control over the circumstances of their dying (autonomy), that they are not duty bound to tolerate every manner of physical insult, pain, and disability (bodily integrity), that sustaining the biological processes of a body that has lost all possibility of human consciousness is disrespectful of the person whose body this once was, and so on.

Such a right is complex, being both a liberty right and an entitlement right. It is a liberty right insofar as it requires others to respect our choices; it is an entitlement right insofar as it obligates others to provide us the necessary resources for living with whatever measure of dignity is possible during dying. These sorts of claims may be more or less strongly asserted, more or less qualified. If, for instance, one were to limit concern for dignity and its desirability solely to self-determination, the "right to die with dignity" would become indistinguishable from the assertion of an unqualified right to suicide. Here one would be operating with a seriously adumbrated concept of "dignity," and making claims very difficult to substantiate, but one would at least be making a claim sufficiently sensible to dispute.

Clearly there cannot be a "right to die" parallel to the "right to live," since the former makes no sense and the latter makes a great deal of sense. Can there, however, be "a right to die with dignity" (understood as a right to a dignified dying process) parallel to and as fundamental as "a right to live with dignity"? There is, I think, a right to die with dignity, but it would be highly misleading to suppose it either parallel to or as fundamental as a right to live with dignity. Rather, the proper relationship between the two, I believe, is that the right to die with dignity is derivable from—or better, but an aspect of—the right to live with dignity. And the right to live with dignity is itself but an aspect of the right to live. Here, in sum, is how it works:

The right to live, if a right at all, is a basic human right.[8] The right to live with dignity is derivable from this basic human right and a theory of justice stipulating what persons are entitled to. There is no symmetry between a right to live and a right to die, nor even between a right to live with dignity and a right to die with dignity. This is because, in the first place, while it makes considerable sense to speak of an existing person's having a fundamental human right to go on living, it makes no sense at all to speak of anyone's having, in any similar or derivative manner, a right to die. Life is something that we might (unjustly) be deprived of by others; no one can "deprive" us of death, nor can anyone guarantee that we have a dying.

The right to live with dignity is therefore secondary to a right to go on living. If we have such a right to live with dignity, then surely it is a right that endures throughout the final phase of living, and that is dying. The right to die with dignity is no more—or less—than the right to live with dignity all the days of our living, until the very end. It is not a separate and distinct right, but part of that right possessed by each human being as a matter of justice. We may, therefore, sensibly speak of a right to die with dignity, so long as we remember that doing so is nothing other than focusing upon our right to live with dignity even while dying. What the right to die with dignity entails we shall consider under the heading of death with dignity as an ideal.

It therefore makes sense to speak of a right to die with dignity, and it is a useful notion for making social policy. What it will do is focus our concern upon the often unique needs and interests of the terminally ill, and remind us that provision needs to be made for meeting these needs to whatever degree doing so is required to preserve the dignity of the dying person and to whatever degree we are committed to allowing persons, as a matter of right, to live with dignity. Which dimensions of human dignity are emphasized will still influence what these policies will be, but that is an altogether legitimate part of a political process.

Medicine and Dying with Dignity

Medicine deals in many different human goods and evils. An adequate exploration of these would go far beyond the scope of this inquiry. But one aspect of medicine essential to every understanding of it is that it attempts to offer people relief from the suffering engendered by disease, injury, and physical impairment. At its most successful, medicine provides relief from such suffering by curing the causes. It is a lesser good, but still a very great one for its beneficiaries, to experience relief from distressing symptoms of inadequately functioning biological systems even where the underlying causes of suffering cannot be cured. In the present context, we can express the aspirations of medicine as being chiefly to promote the human dignity of physical integrity.

But medicine's aspiration to be an enterprise that benefits people is broader than an exclusive focus upon physical well-being can capture. It is persons, in all their complexity, that medical practitioners attempt to benefit. Curing disease, therefore, is not an end in itself. Rather, it is a means to the greater good of benefiting persons suffering from disease. Consequently, in medicine and in nursing there must be concern for more dimensions of human dignity that just physical integrity. There must be concern for the whole person, body and soul as it were, that the complete concept of human dignity attempts to express.

The obvious implication of all this is that medicine cannot be an adequate benefit for persons if it fails to show regard for their dignity as self-conscious, autonomous beings with vital needs to retain consciousness and a sense of self-worth. It is always a difficult and delicate task not to become so enamored of the techniques for combating challenges to bodily integrity that one simultaneously undermines human dignity by disregard for the autonomy and self-respect of patients. Showing due regard for the full range of human dignity is made difficult first by the all too obvious need to address physical functioning, and second, by the increased vulnerability of each of us to having our dignity sabotaged when we are not feeling our best. Disease first, and medicine secondarily, can undermine dignity by making us feel bad, weak and inadequate. Medicine will be of little benefit to us if it fails to respect our needs for dignity in all dimensions. For no one is this more true than for the dying person.

There is, ultimately, no cure for dying. There are things that can be done to help make dying less agonizing than it might otherwise be. Only some of these are the province of medical expertise, for instance, using drugs for pain control. Physicians unable to abandon their commitment to aggressive, curative treatment under all circumstances will not benefit their dying patients but will instead do them great harm. Just one sort of harm that may be done is to deprive the dying of awareness of dying. Another is to close them out of participating in decision-making about what they would like done. Still another is to usurp the opportunity to do those other sorts of things that make dying less agonizing. All these sorts of harm are direct assaults upon the dignity of the dying.

How is death with dignity possible under the conditions in which modern medicine is practiced? The blunt, and often brutal, fact is that all too frequently there is little prospect for dying with dignity. The predominant ethos in medicine is in favor of aggressive treatment to cure disease and disability. Often little accommodation is made to the futility of doing so with the dying. This sort of obsessive need to pursue technological solutions to human tragedies does much to maintain the power of physicians; it does little to respect the dignity of dying persons. Rather, it pointlessly prolongs the dying of the comatose by utilizing sophisticated technologies to maintain biological processes; it keeps children and lovers away from the bedside of the dying; it increases suffering by painful, intrusive treatments with no real benefit; and it badly undermines all aspects of dignity yet retained by the dying.

Eric Cassell has eloquently argued that death with dignity is by and large not possible under the conditions in which modern medicine is practiced. His thesis is that "care of the terminally ill in the United States has changed as the business of dying has shifted from the moral to the technical order." By this he means that as medicine is practiced today, it is not bonds of "sentiment, morality, or conscience" that regulate relationships between persons, but rather notions of the "usefulness of things, based in necessity or expediency," that predominate. Death is now "a technical matter, a failure of technoloy in rescuing the body from a threat to its functioning and integrity."[9]

Those for whom it is especially important to preserve dignity through dying would be well advised to flee the nursing homes and hospitals where medicine is most intensively practiced. If one is very fortunate, there will be a home and a loving family to care for one while he or she dies. Few will be so fortunate. Some few others—mercifully, an increasing number—will be fortunate to experience care intermediate between impersonal hospitals and loving families, care in a hospice or with hospice home care.

The hospice movement is quite self-consciously committed to preserving the dignity of the dying by alleviating debilitating pain, preserving self-esteem, consciousness, and power to make choices, and respecting self-directed choices of the dying. It is an alternative to dying in the domain and under the domination of more traditional medical institutions. Hospice embodies an ethic of personal and professional care that is far from the technological imperatives that concern Cassell. And hospice care, precisely because it uses the best of medical and nursing expertise to assure the physical comfort of the dying and is simultaneously sensitive to a wider range of needs experienced by both those dying and those who love them and will survive them, can often provide care superior to that of those who mean well but are unskilled.[10]

I have emphasized some of the worst aspects of how modern medicine treats the institutionalized dying. It must be confessed that these, no matter how prevalent, are not necessary features of medicine. Technology has not entirely displaced compassion in medicine. There is abundant room within the ethic of medical practice to accommodate the needs of the dying, to preserve their dignity to the greatest extent possible. And there are a great many sensitive practitioners who do so. From the likes of Kübler-Ross, Ciceley Saunders, and Eric Cassell we can learn much about listening to the dying themselves express their desires, and we can learn even more about how to meet the needs of the dying. In this regard, the language of "death with dignity" is again salutary, again useful for urging those changes that will encourage medicine to attend less narrowly to the requirements of preserving physical integrity and more sensitively to respecting all dimensions of human dignity while caring for the dying. Rhetoric and clear thinking alone are very far from sufficient in achieving such changes in institutional medicine, but they are minimally necessary conditions for doing so.

Death with Dignity as an Ideal

Death is the negation of life. Dying is the transition from full living to death. Dying involves many changes, including a progressive loss of personal power, the shedding of all connections to others and the world, and the decline of self-awareness preparatory to the destruction of self. For all this, it is still living, and the requirements for good dying are essentially the same as those for good living: health and emotional stability; meaningful work and personally satisfying activities; freedom from intolerable burdens; love, friendship, and community. If these are the sorts of things we require for living well or with dignity, they will also be the sorts of things we require for dying well or with dignity.

As an ideal for good dying, death with dignity focuses upon several different sorts of interests that dying persons possess. The first of these is, of course, the interest each of us has in maintaining our unique identity and awareness of that identity through self-consciousness. Without this, little else can be of interest to us, and life can have neither dignity nor value for us. Many things short of the loss of consciousness, however, can undermine human dignity, including unbearable pain, and the loss of freedom, health, and self-esteem. Each of these must be protected and preserved for the dying as far as is possible during the inexorable march toward extinction.

But some clear priorities are implied in the caring of the dying by those who would value death with dignity. The first of these is that consciousness and self-awareness are to be preserved as far as possible. Among other things, this requires a very high standard of truth-telling: no lies, no benign deceptions, no paternalistic protection from distasteful revelations, no misleading ambiguities, no silence that shields important information, and no other variations on dissembling are permissible. As Kant forcefully reminded us, few things so undermine human dignity as do lies. By intending to deceive us, the liar wishes us to act on wrongful information. Wise human action is not possible on such a basis, and our very efficacy as autonomous human beings is undermined. There is no dignity in being deliberately deceived. We need only recall the ire and humiliation of Ivan Ilych when confronted by the many denials of his condition that those around him so disingenuously promoted.

Consciousness and self-awareness and rationality are among the requirements for autonomous agency. The second requirement of dying with dignity, or of being treated with dignity while dying, is that one's ability to make choices and implement them be respected. This may require more than merely showing deference to the informed choices made by a dying person. If we have any responsibility for the care of that person, it may require as well that we do what we can to empower him or her to make choices. Just as there is, on the part of physicians, for instance, an obligation to educate their patients, so too there may be an obligation to empower them. We quite rightly expect physicians to do more than treat our ailments; we expect them also to inform us of what they are doing and why, to educate us as to how our bodies work and how they fail to work, to enlighten us about what is happening in our bodies that brought us to them. Both attempts to cure infirmity and to inform ignorance are modes of empowering people; another such mode is to create opportunities in which significant choices about one's own life, or waning of life, can be made.

There are ample opportunities for doing this in the care of the dying. Numerous decisions are made daily about the environment in which the dying are cared for: decisions about diet and routine, about background noise, about whether a radio or TV will be played, about visitors—who, when, how long, etc.—about medication for pain control, about what will be worn, and on and on and on. All too frequently, those most affected by these decisions, the dying themselves, do not participate in making them. Usually this is not because that cannot do so, but rather because they are not expected to do so. This is just one of the reasons that dying in hospital or nursing home is so often devoid of dignity: because in these institutional settings the rules, procedures, routines, and imperatives that predominate have little to do with directly meeting the needs of the dying, and much to do with the convenience and protection of the institution and those who exercise power within it. It is certainly not a bad thing that institutions that serve good purposes be structured so that they survive. But it can be a bad thing if that structuring is done in such a way as to negate some of these good purposes. When this is the case, as it is in hospitals that deny self-determination on the part of the dying, those practices themselves can be resisted, subverted, sometimes even changed. Eliminating such institutional restraints or self-determination would go a great way toward empowering the terminally ill and assuring that dying will be done with dignity.

The two most important aspects of dying with dignity are the maintenance of consciousness and opportunities for self-determination. These in turn require of others absolute candor and integrity with the dying, and efforts not merely to respect self-determination on the part of the dying but to create opportunities for its exercise. Of the other two dimensions of dying with dignity—bodily integrity and self-esteem—there is less to say. Bodily integrity is precisely what dying diminishes and death destroys. The best we can hope for is that dying occur with a minimum of pain and distress, and that others use their skills and compassion to promote this for the dying. It is to be expected that self-esteem will be preserved just to the degree that all these things can be done, that is, insofar as there remain awareness, self-determination and respect for autonomy by others, freedom from unbearable pain and humiliating loss of control, and caring and compassionate treatment by others.

Skeptical Caveats

As an ideal for good dying, death with dignity comes as close as we might hope. It maintains goods of great value and goods greatly valued by the dying. It allows for wide variety in tastes and values for those dying, encouraging them to determine to the greatest degree possible what is required for the maintenance of their dignity. It does not prescribe a set of required attitudes—for example, a benign and accepting regard for death. It offers some clear guidelines to those who would care for the dying on what is required of them. And it offers us the best hope we are likely to find of satisfying the interests of the dying, of survivors, and of morality.

The need to satisfy some requirement of morality for how best to die is a claim of some controversy. There are many grounds on which we might doubt the propriety of imposing expectations upon the dying of how they ought to conduct themselves. One such ground is that to do so is necessarily "sanctimonious cruelty," a kind of moral imperialism on the part of the strong exercised over the weak. The question of justice arises by our having expectations that dying be conducted in a certain fashion, namely, with dignity. Is it fair to impose moral burdens upon the dying precisely at a time when their ability to carry out such obligations is depleted? It might be thought the height of injustice for the yet strong and able to prescribe for the increasingly weak and disabled standards of behavior they must meet.

I think this an altogether legitimate concern, and, if accurate, a telling criticism. But I do not think it is quite right. The moral component of dying with dignity has been distorted by this criticism. It is not that one is morally obligated to die with dignity. Rather, it is morally commendable that one choose to do so. It is quite a separate matter whether those who choose otherwise should be faulted. By and large they surely should not be. Consider the following accounts of persons dying, all of them real persons, recounted as accurately as I can recall:

Betty was 48 years old and in the final stage of metastatic lung cancer. She had had a two to three packs a day cigarette habit for more than thirty years when her disease had been diagnosed six months earlier. Her life had been a hard one. Born into grinding Appalachian poverty, she had been sexually abused by her father at age 12, pregnant by a boyfriend at 14, married at 15, widowed with five children at 21, and had worked at low paying jobs all her life. She birthed seven children, and lived long enough to see three of them die. Death was no stranger to her, and no friend, either. She wanted nothing to do with it.

Betty's attitude toward her dying—a dying more than evident to all about her—was that it was not happening, was not going to happen, and she did not want to know of it. For the first time in her life, others were caring for her, and this was entirely agreeable to her. She was relatively comfortable, warm, had a good bed, and was well fed. She faded very quickly at the end, without ever showing any desire to talk with anyone about dying. She died after two days in a coma.

Betty's two daughters, who had been visiting regularly, were shocked and dismayed by her death. Like their mother, they too did not want to hear about the imminence of death.

Melody was but 23 and suffering an acute form of leukemia. She was terrified of her disease, of the hospital and its procedures, of treatment, and of dying. Her most consistent response to all this terror was tears. She especially implored her mother to protect her from the bone marrow taps—the insertion of a long needle into the pelvis to extract samples of bone marrow—and she became hysterical whenever one of these diagnostic procedures was about to be performed. In the opinion of her physician, she had totally reverted to infantile behavior, and was an extremely difficult patient to manage. The nurses were not much more sympathetic, for they too found her extremely difficult to care for and impossible to speak with about what was happening to her. Only her mother seemed to welcome this behavior, as it gave her the opportunity to exercise a singularly vitriolic tongue on the adequacy of medical care her daughter received. There was no harmony during Melody's dying nor after her death.

Bart was in his early fifties, at the height of his professional power and success as a hospital chaplain, when he died of metastic disease. Four years earlier a malignant tumor had been found on one kidney.

The intervening years saw numerous surgeries, including a colostomy necessitated by a surgical accident during one of his operations. For six months before he died he suffered excruciating pain from spreading cancer in his vertebrae and legs. Yet during this period, Bart accepted only minimal doses of pain killers, because he found that more than a bare minimum did things to his consciousness that he deplored. Mostly what they did was blot it out, either through sleep or through a kind of numbness that prevented him from carrying on conversation. He chose to endure the pain rather than lose his awareness of what was happening and his ability to participate in decision making.

Bart had much to regret. Simultaneous with the progress of his disease, his marriage of more than twenty years was disintegrating, and he was being passed over for promotion in his work. Yet his predominant response was neither bitterness nor withdrawal; he remained open to others, willing to talk about his afflictions but loathe to initiate such conversation, and mostly concerned to put others at ease in his presence. He died in a great deal of pain, but with full consciousness of what was happening.

There is much that might be said about these deaths, more if we knew the people better. But with respect to dying with dignity, only Bart is a viable candidate for this distinction. Betty, with her denial and dependency, does not seem to care about such, and Melody cannot get beyond her terror even to consider such matters. Does this imply that they are somehow morally blameworthy, to be faulted for some significant failing? Surely not. Betty was never privileged to enjoy the means that would have allowed her life to have been characterized as a dignified one; it is hardly to be expected that the end of her living should be so. Dying does not suddenly confer dignity or virtue. But then neither is dying with dignity strictly a matter of character; a great deal depends upon opportunity and good fortune.

I do think it almost always inappropriate to make negative moral judgments about people in extremis, and few conditions are more extreme than dying. Even Melody—whose behavior while dying was offensive to nearly everyone—should be spared the anger that critical moral judgment often embodies. We can only marvel at and admire those singular individuals who choose a response to dying that makes their death easier for others and exemplifies a strength of character that is rare. In the fullest sense of the notion, this is dying with dignity.

Something else to be noted is that abjuring death with dignity does not mean there is no sense in which dying might be good. Betty died the death she chose. She did not wish to die, but having to die, she did not wish to do so in any other fashion. Moreover, she did not die in agonizing pain. These features of her dying might lead one to think there was much about it that was good, just as the one feature of sudden death that inclines to such an evaluation is the freedom from prolonged suffering enjoyed by those who die quickly. It is only if we are prepared to require of good dying that it be as good as dying can be from all perspectives—the deceased's, the surviviors', and judgments made about the deceased—that dying with dignity commends itself to us as the best candidate attainable for ideal dying.

There is a final skeptical caveat to consider, however, and it is a potent one. Alasdair MacIntyre has argued that no notion of "good dying" can make sense anymore, because there are no coherent social structures, rituals, traditions, or institutions within which dying can be given meaning. MacIntyre's is a more radical critique than Cassell's, for while Cassell sees it as a lamentable but remediable feature of medical practice that dying cannot be done well, MacIntyre regards it as a total cultural failing, so severe that nothing less than complete cultural change can make death meaningful, give sense to talk about rights, and so on.[11]

Part of MacIntyre's argument turns on the claim that the only talk of human rights that even makes sense is that which occurs in "the context of a developed and complex form of human practice" (p. 76). Rights belong to individuals "in virtue of their filling certain roles, roles the effective discharge of which is essential to the practice" (p. 77). A practice, in turn, is a rule-governed behavior which specifies its own goods. But in contemporary culture, particularly American, there is no coherent practice that can give rise to the only possible rights, and accordingly no coherent concept of a right way or wrong way to die, of a good or bad death. Instead, what we have is the glorification of the individual, utterly detached from regulative social practices, rituals, and traditions. In this situation, most often known as "individualism," the best one can hope for is perhaps "appropriate death."

I have considerable sympathy with MacIntyre's disenchantment with individualism, less with his praise for social systems that coherently define ideals of good living and good dying through the rigid specification of roles. If the former makes knowing the good difficult or even impossible, the latter makes critical dissent from dominant ideologies of the good and the proper discharge of one's assigned duties so onerous as to exact an enormous price in human freedom. Moreover, there is a good bit to be said for Dworkin's defense of human rights on a basis other than in social systems that rigidly define roles and practices.

But these very large issues of rights and goods, of social roles and freedom, cannot be taken up here. It is enough if we see MacIntyre's challenge to us as being one that suggests that any analysis of good dying in a culture such as ours is necessarily arbitrary and stipulative. It cannot appeal to universally agreed upon standards of goodness or the notions of appropriate living or good dying, because there is no social structure that would make sense of these. If this is so, it undercuts the attempt made here to analyze "death with dignity" and argue that such dying is an appropriate model for good dying.

But I do not think MacIntyre is right. Were he right, we could have no basis on which to admire the likes of Bart, whose dying, while difficult, was conducted with both generosity and great courage on his part. There was a dignity in that dying that commends itself to us, whatever might be the ultimate "incoherence" of our social institutions, traditions, rituals, etc. The notion of dying with dignity explicated here attempts to wend its way between the extremes of unbridled individualism, according to which only a dying person's own choices can define goodness, and the skepticism fostered by MacIntyre's excessive demands for cultural coherence before any aspect of contemporary life can make sense. It attempts to show due, but not excessive, regard for individual choice, and appeal to at least a residue of socially shared values of respect for human dignity. Whether such an analysis succeeds, others must judge.

One limitation, at least, must be acknowledged. However desirable dying with dignity may be for oneself or others, and however admirable it may be from a moral point of view, by itself it will not completely capture all that might be necessary to good dying. Inevitably, much is left to chance, or the fates. That one has a dying at all, and is not just killed, is a matter of fortune frequently beyond anyone's control. That one dies in more or less full possession of mental faculties is also fortuitous. We do not, for instance, even know the cause much less the cure for such a spreading, invidious usurper of human dignity as Alzheimer's disease. And most of all, whether one is born into a time and a place where human dignity is respected at all and conditions are favorable for living with dignity is completely a matter of chance.

No doubt for these and many similar reasons, the ancient Greeks were of the opinion that we could not know whether a person's life had been a happy—or, we might say, a dignified—one until it was over. Only then could we know whether the combination of uncontrollable circumstance and self-chosen character had created a life with happiness and dignity. This much has not changed, nor will it.

Part II
Choosing Death

INTRODUCTION TO PART II

What emerges most strongly from our long journey through numerous conceptual confusions and value conflicts explored in Part I is the centrality of concern with human dignity that any extended reflection on
death and dying must address. A focus on human dignity arose toward
the end of exploring connections between death, good, and evil; from
henceforth it will be a constant presence.

Part II takes up the issues of how to understand suicide, whether
there is a right to suicide and the nature of such a possible right, autonomous refusals of life-sustaining treatment, and procedures and criteria
for allowing avoidable death for persons who cannot themselves choose
it but for whom such a choice might well be best. All of these fall under
the rubric of *Choosing Death*.

Not only does human dignity become central under this heading; our
focus also shifts essentially from private value choices about how to regard our own deaths to questions about public policy on suicide and euthanasia. For example, chapter seven begins with philosophical concerns
about the concept of suicide and moves, by the end of chapter eight, to
consideration of the implications of the intervening analysis for what
should be public policy on suicide. Similarly, chapters nine and ten
begin with very personal, individual dilemmas of severely ill or injured
persons and go on to consider how fair and decent treatment of these persons implies a number of desirable policies in medicine specifically and society generally.

Suicide is vexing from almost any point of view. The first task I under-
take in Part II is to bring some conceptual clarity to the concept of suicide (chapter seven). But this turns out to be not at all simple, since the
concept of suicide seems often to be inextricably bound up with moral evaluations of it. By any measure, however otherwise we might wish it, 'suicide' is a value-laden term.

In the end, therefore, I argue that it is much preferable to view the concept of suicide as an "open-textured" notion, rather than one for which
necessary and sufficient conditions of applicability can be specified.
So regarding suicide introduces an unavoidable element of both conceptual
and moral relativism, for which deaths we will count as suicide turns out
to depend very strongly on the purposes we bring to our evaluation. For
different persons with different interests—for example, priests, psychiatrists, coroners, and insurance agents—the assessment of which deaths
will be counted as suicide can be expected to vary considerably.

The most interesting question we might ask about suicide, I think, is
not the question of how precisely to define "suicide," but the question of

whether persons can be said to have a right—especially a fundamental right—to choose to end their own lives (chapter eight). Merely asking this question puts the phenomenon of suicide in a light different from the usual one in which suicide is regarded as a problem to be prevented.

Three different bases are explored for grounding a right to suicide. The first of these is that each person's life belongs to oneself alone, and, like other property one might own, it can be disposed of as the owner pleases. The second ground is that exercising the power to kill oneself is an exercise of liberty, a right of autonomy possessed by all competent moral agents. Finally, it might be supposed that the right to kill oneself is simply fundamental, on a level with a right to life itself, or freedom of thought and expression, and so on.

The first two of these foundations rest on shifting sand and will not bear up under the heavy burden of moral justification that choices for self-inflicted death impose on one. The last is more adequate—at least it is no more inadequate than other claims to fundamental human rights— but it needs careful qualification.

M. Pabst Battin has argued strongly that "we have a right to suicide (if and when we do) because it is constitutive of human dignity." I think this is a fundamentally sound claim, but one that needs extensive testing and careful clarification. When this is done, I argue, it turns out that as basic as the right to suicide may be, the occasions on which it is justifiably exercised are very few.

One of the most severe challenges possible to a right to choose death is presented by Dax Cowart, who at age 26 was very severely burned, and who suffered more than a year of excruciatingly painful treatments that he never wanted (chapter nine). But Cowart was caught in a generally well-intentioned medical system in which the practioners regarded it as their moral obligation to sustain his life, however little he may have desired it. The case for treating him against his will, as well as the argument for not treating him, in accord with his seemingly competent and informed choice to reject life-sustaining care, both raise extremely complex and subtle issues of morality. Among these are issues concerning the autonomy rights of competent persons, the obligations of medical professionals, what really constitutes patient benefit and good medical care, paternalism, the value of life, and the obligations of patients.

But as with all real cases, the disagreements are not solely moral: much in the very description of the situation is in dispute. Factual disagreement occurs over whether Cowart really does prefer death to treatment and the life continuing treatment might give him, whether his caregivers consistently intend the best for him, whether Cowart has a competent person's sense of himself, what precisely he can be said to suffer, and so on.

In the final analysis, I think, Cowart's fundamental right to choose for himself whether to go on with life must be respected, even if this means he will die. In his case—and in all relevantly similar cases, of which there are many in medicine—human dignity is enhanced by respecting a competent person's informed choice to die rather than endure even life-prolonging treatment when in that person's judgment such prolonged life is not a worthwhile outcome of unduly burdensome treatments.

This conclusion raises a special problem for what choices should be made in similar circumstances for persons who cannot make their own choices (chapter ten). On the face of it, we do not want to say that impaired human beings have fewer rights than the (temporarily) able-bodied and sound of mind; yet how can we respect the rights of those unable themselves to assert and exercise their rights? This issue is raised with special poignancy for Joseph Saikewicz, who while severely retarded and a ward of the state, was found to be suffering very acute leukemia at age 66. Who has the right to decide on Mr. Saikewicz's behalf what shall be done? And as important, according to what criteria shall an authorized decision-maker choose?

Increasingly, these questions have been decided in courts of law—and not just for never-competent persons such as Saikewicz, but also for once-competent persons such as Edna Marie Leach, who had quite clearly expressed her desire not to be sustained on life support in the event she lost the capacity to assert as much when it might actually be needed.

I argue that it makes a difference whether one has never been (and never will be) able to participate in decision-making, or whether one has irretrievably lost a once realized capacity. Moreover, we need a far more refined notion of "substituted judgment" than courts have generally invoked to protect the disabled, and a clearer notion of whether it is rights or interests that most need protection.

Sorting all this out and applying it to Joseph Saikewicz is vitally important. But in the end we are left with the irrevocable tragedy of a life that was less than it might have been, and that ended worse than it should have. In this regard, there is the threat that Joseph Saikewicz is a woeful everyman of the near future. But that future is one that, with enough clear thinking, goodwill, and vigorous struggle, need not be.

VII

SUICIDE
CHOOSING SELF-INFLICTED DEATH

> For who would bear the whips and scorns
> of time,
> The oppressor's wrong, the proud man's
> contumely,
> The pangs of despised love, the law's
> delay,
> The insolence of office, and the spurns
> That patient merit of the unworthy takes,
> When he himself might his quietus make
> With a bare bodkin?
>
> William Shakespeare
> *Hamlet*

> There is but one truly serious philosophical
> problem, and that is suicide.
>
> Albert Camus
> *The Myth of Sisyphus*

Camus is almost certainly mistaken in making such a bold claim, but he does succeed in drawing our attention to a topic too little attended by philosophers. He is mistaken both because suicide is not chiefly a philosophical problem (it is many other sorts of problems, including psychological, sociological, political, and so on) and because there are many other "truly serious philosophical problems." Nonetheless, as a philosophical problem, suicide divides roughly into two sorts of concerns. On the one hand, there is the central philosophical task of conceptual analysis, according to which we seek to understand just what is meant by "suicide." This involves analysis of the uses of the word "suicide" to discern its meaning, or, equally often with this particular concept, a stipulative definition of what "suicide" will be taken to mean. On the other hand, a major philosophical task is to evaluate the morality of suicide. These distinct tasks have not always been clearly separated, and much confusion has resulted from their being conflated.

One would hope that the difference between identifying an act as one of suicide and evaluating that act as a morally worthy or unworthy act would be clear. Such clarity may not be altogether possible, however, if our very understanding of "suicide" has built into it a number of morally evaluative notions, as seems often to be the case. The most frequently offered dictionary definition of suicide is "self-murder," and of murder, "morally wrong killing." By parity of reasoning, therefore, the very definition of suicide entails its moral wrongness. A more neutral definition of suicide might be "self-killing," as fewer evaluative questions are begged by characterizing an act as one of killing rather than one of murder.[1]

This bias built into dictionary definitions of suicide is but a reflection of a far deeper cultural prejudice, even a taboo. In the West, the most vigorous condemnation of suicide began with Augustine, who was at pains to deter the rather too enthusiastic seeking after death and eternal salvation that ever more powerful cults were having upon the newly respectable and established religion of Christianity. So successful was Augustine's campaign that soon the Church adopted an antisuicide stance as dogmatic as anything held by those who had formerly sought suicide as the path to salvation. The state followed in due course, so that in England, for instance, the punishment for suicide was public denigration of the corpse, burial at a crossroads with a stake driven through one's heart (as with witches), and confiscation of all one's property by the Crown. Those who attempted but failed at suicide fared even worse: in addition to all of the above, they were hanged![2]

Analyses more careful and thorough than dictionary definitions have not always succeeded in escaping the taint of prejudging the morality of suicide by defining it as immoral. Thus in the long tradition of Catholic moral theology, suicide has been understood to be "morally wrongful self-killing," and those self-killings that were not regarded as "morally wrongful" were explained away as not suicides because they occurred at the command of God or as heroic self-sacrifices, and the like. "Martyrdom" and "self-sacrificing death," however deliberate, intentional, or chosen, were not regarded as suicides because they were regarded as commendable and it is inconceivable that suicide could be commendable.

This long history in the West of conflating the definition with the evaluation of suicide is the first reason that it is now very difficult to put forth a morally neutral definition of suicide. There is further a second difficulty in doing so, and that is that the concept of suicide, in any culture, may be so complex as not to admit of definition through the specification of necessary and sufficient conditions for its application. Suicide is, after all, perhaps above all, a human action, and the analysis of human action involves some of the most elusive and controversial concepts of all. Where suicide is under consideration, these include at least the following highly problematical concepts: knowledge, intention, desire, and will; causation, compulsion, coercion, and a distinction between doing and suffering; voluntary, nonvoluntary, involuntary, and the principle of double effect; and many more.

Both because of the historical tendency to conflate defining and evaluating suicide and because of the philosophical complexity of the many concepts inherent in understanding acts of suicide, one might despair of attaining any clear understanding of what suicide is, much less of how to go about reasonably evaluating suicides.

But the situation is not as hopeless as this implies. Philosophical analysis offers more tools for understanding than defintions that exhaustively specify necessary and sufficient conditions for the application of a concept, and moral evaluation can proceed on a basis other than by building into the very definition of an action its moral value. Notwithstanding the above difficulties, then, the task before us is, first, to attain some reasonable understanding of what we mean by "suicide," and, second, to find a path through the labyrinth of conflicting moral intuitions that will enable us to evaluate with sensitivity choices for self-inflicted death.

Suicide Case Studies

The following cases will be useful references for both attempting to understand the concept of suicide and evaluating the morality of suicide. They will not suffice to say everything one might want to say about these matters, but they ought to be adequate to the task at hand.

Case 1: Anne Marleybone

> Anne Marleybone was doing what she enjoyed doing most: flying her two-seat Piper Cub. It was a gorgeous, clear day, and Anne was feeling wonderful. But then the tail section of her plane, without warning, began to break up. Anne realized that soon she would lose all control of the craft. Fortunately, she was equipped with a parachute. But before bailing out, Ms. Marleybone made some quick calculations. It appeared that if she bailed out, the plane would likely crash in a schoolyard filled with children playing. But if she stayed with the plane and attempted to guide it to a cornfield a block away, she would certainly die. Anne Marleybone stayed with her plane. (Postscript: The plane crashed in the schoolyard, injuring sixteen children, killing three children and Anne Marleybone.)[3]

Case 2: Linda Ault

The following account of the death of Linda Marie Ault is quoted in its entirety from the *New York Times*, February 7, 1968:

> Linda Marie Ault killed herself, policemen said today, rather than make her dog Beauty pay for her night with a married man.
> " 'I killed her. I killed her. It's just like I killed her myself,' " a detective quoted her grief-stricken father as saying.
> " 'I handed her the gun. I didn't think she would do anything like that.' "

The 21-year-old Arizona State University coed died in a hospital yesterday of a gunshot wound in the head.

The police quoted her parents, Mr. and Mrs. Josept Ault, as giving this account:

" 'Linda failed to return home from a dance in Tempe Friday night. On Saturday she admitted she had spent the night with an Air Force Lieutenant.' "

The Aults decided on a punishment that would "wake Linda up." They ordered her to shoot the dog she had owned about two years.

On Sunday, the Aults and Linda took the dog into the desert near their home. They had the girl dig a shallow grave. Then Mrs. Ault grasped the dog between her hands, and Mr. Ault gave his daughter a .22-caliber pistol and told her to shoot the dog.

Instead, the girl put the pistol to her right temple and shot herself.

The police said there were no charges that could be filed against the parents except possibly cruelty to animals.[4]

Case 3: George Angeles

A man, whom we will call George Angeles, killed himself and left the following note behind:

Dear Betty:
    I hate you.
       love,
          George[5]

Case 4: Leslie Tharp

Leslie Tharp died on October 31, 1981. He was at the time an Associate Professor in the Philosophy Department of the University of Illinois at Chicago Circle, and a man widely respected for his significant contributions to logic and philosophy.

Leslie received a B.S. degree in 1962 from the Mathematics Department of MIT. Three years later he received a Ph.D. from the department after writing a dissertation on constructive set theory. He stayed on as an instructor until 1967, and then joined the Logic Group at Rockefeller University. . .

Those who knew Leslie Tharp will remember him as a quiet, modest, and gentle man. He was deeply serious about his work, but he never lost a sparkling appreciation of how ridiculous academic life can be. He grew up on a small farm in North Dakota and sometimes thought it curious that he ever left. Leslie's students will remember him as a gifted and dedicated teacher. Though severely self-critical, he was always generous and supportive in his dealings with them.

Throughout his life Leslie suffered from severe clinical depresssion. His attacks became ever more crippling in recent years. He tried numerous forms of therapy without relief, and eventually became convinced that his condition was incurable. He then decided to end his life. His suicide was an act of desperation, but not of panic. It was carefully planned in advance. Until the end Leslie never ceased to think of others.[6]

Case 5: John Rarrick

John Rarrick had been seriously depressed, on and off, for most of his life since age 14. When he was 17, he nearly died in an auto accident when the car he was driving at 80 mph slid off a rain-slicked road and hit a tree. At 19 he nearly drowned when, swimming in the ocean, he found himself too far from shore to return. Only a passing sailboat saved his life then. At 24 an overdose of alcohol and barbiturates nearly killed him, and did put him into a two-week long coma. After this he began intensive psychotherapy, but his depressions recurred. At 29 he died of asphyxiation when, inebriated, he fell asleep in his car while the engine was running in an enclosed garage.[7]

Case 6: Samson

And Samson said unto the lad that held him by the hand, Suffer me that I may feel the pillars whereupon the house standeth, that I may lean upon them.

Now the house was full of men and women; and all the lords of the Philistines were there; and there were upon the roof about three thousand men and women, that beheld while Samson made sport.

And Samson called unto the Lord, and said, O Lord God, remember me, I pray thee, and strengthen me, I pray thee, only this once, O God, that I may be at once avenged of the Philistines for my two eyes.

And Samson took hold of the two middle pillars upon which the house stood, and on which it was borne up, of the one with his right hand, and of the other with his left.

And Samson said, Let me die with the Philistines. And he bowed himself with all his might; and the house fell upon the lords, and upon all the people that were therein. So the dead which he slew at his death were more than they which he slew in his life.[8]

Case 7: Marcellus

Marcellus was a Circumcellion, a particularly fanatical subgroup of the zealous Donatists, an early Christian sect. For Donatists, the surest route to salvation was martyrdom, and they welcomed it. Circumcellions went several steps further, advocating and practicing suicide in the effort to achieve martyrdom.

Marcellus had a dream one night that he interpreted as a revelation that "his time was at hand." Insecure of salvation, and eager for martyrdom, he proceeded to the nearest highway, where he stopped the first Roman magistrate coming down the road. Raising his sword, he said to the magistrate: "Kill me, or be killed." The Roman obliged Marcellus.[9]

Case 8: Mass Suicide

M. Pabst Battin gives the following account of mass suicide:

During the Second World War, the directress of an orthodox Jewish girls' school in a Nazi-occupied city came to understand that her girls, ranging in age from twelve to eighteen, had been kept from extermina-

tion in order to provide sexual services for the Gestapo. When the Gestapo announced its intention to avail themselves of these services—
ordering the directress to see that the girls were washed and prepared
for defloration by "pure aryan youth"—she called an assembly and distributed poison to each of the students, teachers, and herself. The ninety-
three maidens, as they have come to be called, swallowed the poison, re-
cited a final prayer, and died undefiled.[10]

Case 9: Harry Parkinson

Harry Parkinson had taught in the public schools nearly all of his
adult life, ever since discharge from the Merchant Marine at age 25. He
worked his way up through the ranks of physical education teacher, football coach, vice-principal (for discipline), to principal of a high school,
where he served until retirement at age 65.

Retirement was difficult for Harry. He had few interests outside of his
work, and few friends that he cared to spend time with (or who, it appeared, cared to spend time with Harry). When at 67 he was found to
have a serious but treatable blood disease, Harry regarded it as a death sentence. The oncologist's assurance that Harry could be expected to live several good years with this disease did little to cheer him. He gave only
perfunctory cooperation to a course of chemotherapy, and when hospital-
ized for his rapidly deteriorating physical condition, resisted blood transfusions. To the oncologist, consulting psychiatrist, his wife of thirty years,
and both his adult children, Harry had but one thing to say: "I just want
out."

The psychiatrist thought Harry was emotionally blocked, paralyzed by
fear, and depressed. He did not think Mr. Parkinson suffered a "mental illness." His wife thought he was "just being Harry."

Four months after diagnosis, Harry Parkinson died as a consequence
of his rapidly spreading disease.[11]

Case 10: Betty Blue

Betty Blue was 83 years old and for the last five years of her life had
been resident in a state-run nursing home. Most of her life she had been
a ballet dancer, then the head of a dance school of considerable regional re-
pute. But now she had outlived her husband of more than half a century, most of her friends, and, most tragically of all for her, her only daughter. Moreover, Betty suffered diminished memory and increasing mental
confusion, severe joint pain from rheumatoid arthritis, circulatory problems that had necessitated the amputation of her right leg above the
knee and that were threatening the same to her left leg, impaired hearing, and advanced glaucoma. Recent intestinal difficulties and discomfort
strongly implied tumor growth, but Betty's frailty prevented the explora-
tory surgery needed to confirm as much.

Betty was still able to move about in a wheelchair, and was for the
most part mentally alert. One evening she made her way to the cleaner's
closet and stole a full liter bottle of liquid Drano. She took it back to her
room, where she wrote the following note before drinking the Drano
and dying:

I have lived a full life. It has not been without pain, disappointment and tragedy, but on the whole I am satisfied. I had a good husband, a loving daughter, creative and meaningful work, and many good friends. One cannot hope for more than that. But that is all behind me now, and I see no point in going on down this path that promises only pointless pain and increasing disability. My only regret is that I am forced down this path alone; I would rather others help me, and spare me this final indignity. But I prefer this death now to the greater indignities of this life.

love to all,
Betty Blue[12]

Defining Suicide

Despite the earlier noted difficulties in defining suicide—that it comes to us as an already morally loaded term, and that it involves a number of highly complex concepts—we do not yet have sufficient reason to think it not possible to provide an analysis or not worthwhile to do so. Indeed, for a variety of very different purposes, to be noted presently, it is essential that we be very clear about what we will and will not regard as suicide. We shall proceed, then, by examining a number of significant attempts to provide a compelling definition of suicide.

To define an act as one of suicide requires the identification of a set of conditions that when met will be jointly necessary and sufficient for the application of the concept. Such attempts have historically covered a broad range of conditions, and have varied from being very "loose" and "permissive" (i.e., allowing many acts that result in the death of a person to be counted as suicide), to being very "tight" and "narrow." At the narrow end of the spectrum are those definitions of suicide which insist upon the centrality of a person's intending to bring about his or her death in a deliberate and active manner. Thus Richard Brandt, a contemporary philosopher, regards suicide

as doing something which results in one's death, either from the intention of ending one's life or the intention to bring about some other state of affairs (such as relief from pain) which one thinks it certain or highly probable can be achieved only by means of death. . . .[13]

For all of its "narrowness," in insisting upon a clear intention to destroy oneself, notice how encompassing Brandt's notion of suicide is. Virtually all of the cases given above qualify as suicides under his definition, with the possible exception of John Rarrick, who, while clearly of a suicidal bent, does not allow us to judge precisely his intentions in the garage at the time of his death. But even Anne Marleybone—not a suicide for those who think motive crucial—is so on Brandt's account, since, by staying with her plane rather than bailing out, she could not be regarded as other than choosing, quite deliberately and intentionally, her own death as the price of sparing some children. Her intention "to bring about some other state of affairs" (saving the children), achievable "only by means of death," makes her a suicide on Brandt's criteria.

A still narrower definition of suicide could be attained if it were insisted that only one's primary intention is relevant for an act to be one of suicide. This would eliminate Anne Marleybone as a suicide, since clearly she did not want to die so much as she wanted to spare the children. On the other hand, it might also eliminate Linda Ault, George Angeles, Samson, and even the Ninety-three Maidens from being regarded as suicides. Ault and Angeles acted with some ambivalence, but with clear hostility toward others. This is all we know of George Angeles, but it may well be that his intention to hurt his wife was primary. Linda Ault's case is more complex (or at least we know more to warrant this judgment). Among other things, she must have felt intense conflict, including some mixture of guilt, shame, rage, and impotence. That she did violence to herself, rather than her parents, may have been the only way she could find to strike out at them. And that could have been something she wanted even more than death.

But Samson and the Ninety-three Maidens are not candidates for suicide on even the most narrow requirement that one's primary intention be self-destruction. Samson intended vengeance and the destruction of his enemies. In this he succeeded spectacularly. The Ninety-three Maidens intended to remain undefiled, and they too succeeded in the only way available to them. By any other measure, deliberately pulling a building down upon one's self, or ingesting what one knows to be a deadly dose of poison, is certainly suicide.

But as it happens, broad definitions of suicide are hardly more satisfactory than narrow ones. Sociologists, following in Durkheim's footsteps, have been most drawn to a definition that requires no more than "knowingly" doing something risky that results in death. Psychiatrists, following Karl Menninger, have sometimes taken this even further afield from any conscious state of mind (deliberation, intention, knowledge, etc.) and regarded any behavior that is harmful as suicidal, and any that results in death as suicide. On such an account as this, mere living is suicidal, since all living inevitably brings us closer to death, and all dying is suicide.[14]

One of the most careful analyses of suicide, one that seeks to wend its way through the deficiencies of definitions either too narrow or too broad and at the same time leave the moral evaluation of suicide largely an open question, is Tom Beauchamp's. Beauchamp sets forth three requirements for suicide. These are that

1. a person *intentionally* brings about his or her death;
2. the person is *not coerced* by others to suicide;
3. death is caused in circumstances *specifically arranged* for the purpose of bringing about his or her death.[15]

On this account, Anne Marleybone is not a suicide, and we do not know about John Rarrick. That much seems intuitively agreeable. But further, Harry Parkinson and the Ninety-three Maidens are not suicides either, and that is somewhat more problematical. Harry Parkinson intended to die, we may suppose, and he was certainly not coerced by others to do so. Yet he cannot be said to have "specifically arranged" the circumstances that caused his death. He might, as it were, "have taken advantage" of circumstances to let a deadly disease do what he might otherwise have chosen to do, but this is far short of "specifically arranging" conditions for the purpose of bringing about death. If the intention to die is clear (and here Harry Parkinson is not the best case but will suffice), how much does it really matter that a person arranges the means to bring death about? Won't it do as well to take advantage of circumstances that could be, but are not, avoided?

The Maidens are not suicides, because what they did they were coerced into doing by others: broadly speaking, by the Nazis, and more immediately, by their headmistress. The Nazis did not directly command their deaths; they simply offered as the only alternative a fate presumably worse than death. But the headmistress did demand that they die. In the name of religious principle, and using all her authority and power to influence the girls, she provided them poison and insisted it was both in their interest and their obligation to take it. However benignly intended, what she did and the circumstances in which she did it go far beyond encouragement and constitute coercion. But for all this, can it be right, as Beauchamp would seem committed to saying, to regard these ninety-three girls as not suiciding? While a maximum degree of freedom from coercion may be required for moral responsibility, it is not so necessary for choice itself. What is at stake here is not the rightness or wrongness of their choice, but whether choice is possible where coercion is present. For these girls, as for Candide, it would seem to be so. Coercion does not disqualify one's choice from being suicide.[16]

Morally loaded, narrow, broad, and careful compromise definitions of suicide have all failed to provide definitions that will enable us to agree on whether certain difficult cases of a person's involvement in doing something to bring about his or her death will be regarded as suicide. Two observations are in order. First, it might be useful to reflect on why we think a definition of suicide is necessary, and second, it would be useful to consider whether the concept of suicide can better be understood by an approach that abjures identifying necessary and sufficient conditions for its application.

The Uses of a Definition
of Suicide

Why then do we need to be clear about the concept of suicide, however murky it may be and difficult to get a grasp on? Apart from the obvious desirability of being able to understand an important phenomenon better, there are several very practical uses to which some notion of suicide is put. A tragic automobile accident in which the lone driver was burned to death after his car collided with a bridge abutment became something else altogether when the coroner's investigator discovered that he was driving with an open gallon of gasoline between his legs and smoking a cigarette as he ran into the abutment.[17] In this case, the Coroner's Office, the county's mortality statistics, the life insurance company that refused indemnity (never mind the double indemnity clause for accidental death), and the man's relatives were all deeply affected by the pronouncement of death by suicide rather than accidental death. And since this man belonged to a church that regarded suicide as a mortal sin, so too did his reputation in that community greatly decline.

Other quite practical interests are affected by the decision to label a death suicide. Sociologists, for instance, need to know what warrants this judgment in order to study the incidence of suicide in a community. Psychiatrists need to understand its psychodynamics in order to treat patients. And all of us with a commitment to reducing death by suicide need some understanding of just what this is in order to design community programs of crisis intervention and suicide prevention.

Not all these interests are equally compelling or serious. From a moral point of view, greatest concern might be shown for those persons in such a state that suicide is contemplated, and for those left behind to grieve after a suicide occurs. The latter especially have a difficult time understanding, accepting, or reconciling themselves to the loss through suicide of someone they love. There is a very special difficulty in grasping that someone we love has chosen death over life. Here grief is laced with guilt, with a sense of having failed someone we love. And often this is so even where the dead person means us no harm, acts toward us with no hostility.

Underlying these different interests and purposes in being clear about what counts as suicide is our need to morally evaluate human actions, and the special difficulties of doing so for those actions on the margin of life. Death by self-inflicted means, by suicide, provokes in us as profound and varied a set of emotional reactions as anything human beings do. Beyond sorrow, typical emotional responses to the suicide of someone we care about are guilt, anger, fear, and a sense of personal threat. These emotions often underlie the harsh judgments we make about the morality of suicide, precisely because one of the ways civilized persons have of responding to such a sense of personal threat is to condemn the threatener with the language of morality. While such may be preferable to more conventional and explicit violence, it still falls far short of a rational and reasoned response. And for all the difficulty there may be in making reasonable moral judgments about suicide, it is necessary and desirable to do so. But for the present it must remain an open question as to whether the labeling of an act as one of suicide is a useful aid in the legitimate enterprise of morally evaluating human actions. A decision about this must await greater clarity on what to count as suicide.

And we still do not know what acts to count as suicide, what not. I think at this point, however, we shall not make progress by continuing to look for definitive markers of suicide. This is because, however much we would want it otherwise, there are none. Not only is there no precise set of features the presence of which is sufficient for identifying a death as a suicide, but there is not even one such feature that is universally necessary to suicide—not an intention or a desire to die, not choice, not even the achievement of death itself. This is to suggest that we should abandon all attempts to define suicide, and consider instead a different approach to understanding the concept.

Criteria for Suicide

Our error so far has been to suppose that any definition could capture a phenomenon as diverse, as variously motivated, with such very different states of mind, occurring in such different circumstances by such varied means, as sometimes vague, and as most often baffling and mysterious, as suicide. Suicide is an open-textured concept, lacking precise boundaries, but not lacking coherence. Our best understanding of what is and is not to count as suicide is likely to come when we see that there are criteria for suicide, but no set of specifications that are invariable. This is to say that there are varying combinations of characteristics of events legitimately labeled suicide, but no particular set of them that is sufficient and no one that is necessary for a death to be suicide. This allows that while certain deaths will be transparently clear as suicide, others will be highly disputable and borderline. For different purposes, we might well select different combinations of characteristics present in suicide, use different criteria out of the frequently fluid set available.

In the case studies set forth, there is no one feature present in all by virtue of which each is a suicide. Nor is there a specific combination of features that makes each a suicide (or lacking these, not a suicide). There are clear, even paradigm cases—Linda Ault, Leslie Tharp, Betty Blue—and marginal, arguable, borderline cases—John Rarrick, Harry Parkinson, and others perhaps. Not even death itself is a necessary feature of those acts we might call suicide, as we can imagine the following case, which we would be prepared to call suicide even though death does not occur: a man places his head in a stamping machine, which crushes his skull, but "only" destroys enough brain capacity to render him permanently vegetative but not dead even by brain-death criteria. Twenty years later he dies of congestive heart failure. Is he a suicide? That a case can be made that he is indicates just how variable are the combinations of criteria for suicide.

Among the criteria for suicide are death; death caused by actions or behavior of the deceased (active or passive);

> that the deceased wanted, desired, or wished death; that the deceased intended, chose, decided, or willed to die; that the deceased knew that death would result from his behavior; that the deceased was responsible for his death.[18]

And this list is not exhaustive, merely illustrative of the range of considerations relevant to the specification of acts of suicide. Accordingly, psychiatrists are likely to have little difficulty in seeing John Rarrick as a suicide. His long history of depression and suicidal behavior, of near death in increasingly suspicious circumstances, indicates a personality disposed to self-destruction that finally accomplishes a long sought after goal. But coroners, who require much more explicit and public evidence of precise intention to die before labeling a dead person a suicide, must give the benefit of doubt to Mr. Rarrick.

Neither psychiatrists nor coroners are going to regard Anne Marleybone or Samson as suicides, but all who emphasize the centrality of intention, and do not scruple about primary and secondary intentions or doctrines of "double effect," will have little difficulty in doing so. Durkheim, for instance, might well include both Marleybone and Samson in his category of "altruistic suicide." Those who insist upon the importance of the deceased's having used an active, not a passive, means to bring about death may disqualify Harry Parkinson from the class of suicides. On some accounts not even Marcellus is a suicide, as he does not kill himself, however much he maneuvers to coerce another to kill him. And so on.

However, several of the deaths among our case studies will not be counted as suicides by some persons, not because of doubts about agency, intention, desire, means, or the like, but just because these persons will insist that nothing must be regarded as a suicide that is not certainly morally wrong. Hence some other label must be found for Marleybone and Samson, perhaps for Marcellus and the Ninety-three Maidens, even for Harry Parkinson and Betty Blue. But this is, I have already suggested, a mistake, for it is far better to separate the criteria for identifying an act as one of suicide from those for evaluating such acts. Such conflation as this, in the cases of Marleybone, Samson, Marcellus, the Ninety-three Maidens, Parkinson, and Blue, simply muddies waters already murky.

Morally Evaluating Suicide

And yet, there are more reasons than cultural bias and conceptual complexity for being unable completely to separate criteria for identifying and evaluating suicides. These tasks are different, but they do overlap. For instance, in deciding whether a death is a suicide it is often important to know the deceased's intentions. But intentions are also very relevant for evaluating acts in many moral systems. Thus if one believes both that suicide must be an intentional choice for death and that an intention to die is always morally wrong, it will not be possible ever to separate characterizing an act as suicide and judging it morally unworthy. Suicide is simply wrong.

The overlap of the criteria for identifying and evaluating suicide, however, need not result in the errors of the previous paragraph. It seems to me there are two errors of considerable consequence. The first of these is the smuggling back into our understanding of what is useful for identifying suicide the conviction that there is some necessary feature in all suicides, here specified as "an intentional choice for death," and not a variable set of criteria. The second is the very much more controversial supposition that a useful, categorical judgment about the moral propriety of suicide is possible.

If one is persuaded that suicide is identifiable by a varying set of criteria, different subsets of which are legitimately used for different purposes, one could avoid both errors. The very recognition of the need for criteria rather than necessary and sufficient defining conditions for suicide avoids the error of supposing any single feature is necessary to suicide. Furthermore, this recognition ought to go a long way toward diminishing the temptation to offer categorical and absolutist judgments on suicide. It avoids such judgments by impressing upon us just how variable are the intentions, desires, and wishes of those who suicide; how diverse are the circumstances in which death is "chosen"; how different the consequences for survivors and society, and so on. Given this enormous diversity in all the categories available for moral evaluation, and the lack of any single feature or set of features that defines suicide as such, it is no longer even plausible to suppose one judgment about the morality of suicide makes sense.

Consider just some of the more obvious variability in choices for death that are plausible suicides. Choosing to expedite death where death is in any case imminent, necessary, or assured (Betty Blue?) is significantly different from those suicides in which death will not otherwise occur, where death is an alternative to life of indefinite duration (Leslie Tharp). Similarly, there is a vast gulf between those choices for self-inflicted death that are directed at harming others (George Angeles?) and those that benefit others (Anne Marleybone); between those that are mad (no cases given) and those that are rational (arguably, a majority of the case studies); between those that are impulsive (Linda Ault) and those that are carefully planned (Leslie Tharp); between those that are responses to unbearable suffering (Betty Blue) and those that are cowardly flights from hardship (Harry Parkinson?); between suicides that are cries for help gone too far (Alvarez's view of Sylvia Plath) and suicides quite unambiguously engineered (Samson, Marcellus); and so on.

So variable are the types of suicide that one suspects it is only plausible to offer a categorical judgment about the (im)morality of suicide if one has nurtured himself or herself on "an inadequate diet of examples."[19] Be this as it may, there has been no lack of sweeping condemnation of suicide in the history of thought and culture. My hope is that the approach taken here, of arguing the impossibility of essentialist definitions of suicide, and inviting reflection on how variable actual suicides are in every dimension, will finesse the need for refuting these sweeping judgments one by one.[20]

Once we give up an essentialist definition of suicide, it should be possible to see not only how sweeping judgments about the morality of suicide as such are misbegotten, but also how a great many other generalizations about suicide are false. Thus no more than that all suiciders are "sinners" is it the case that all have "diseased minds" and are "mentally ill."[21] Nor is it the case that all suicide attempts are "cries for help," and that successful suicides are attempts gone (unintentionally) too far. Other myths of suicide, born of the tendency to excessive generalization, include the notions that successfully preventing a suicide will deter that person from ever trying again; that would-be suicides are grateful for being "rescued"; that intervention to prevent suicide is always morally justified; that a psychotherapist's obligation is always to prevent a client's suiciding, and so on.

To suggest that no categorical judgment about the morality of suicide is possible is far from suggesting that no moral assessments of particular suicides are possible or even that there are no generally valid principles by which such judgments can be made. But it is to suggest that simply deciding to characterize an act as a suicide is not particularly helpful to a moral assessment of the act. Being able to pin the label "suicide" on a death does virtually nothing to inform us in any reasonable way whatever whether that death was good or bad, right or wrong, reasonable or unreasonable, rational or irrational, and so on. About such deaths as we are certain or even inclined to call suicide, two far more specific questions must be asked if we are to make any reasonable evaluation of their morality. These are:

1. Does this person choose to die?

2. Does this person have compelling, good reasons for choosing to die?

Together, these questions amount to asking whether it is morally permissible for a person to choose death and do what is necessary to bring his or her own death about. Answering the first of the questions is important for several reasons. I have already argued (chapter six) that respect for human dignity is vital, and that a central element in human dignity is the exercise of autonomy. An important part of one's autonomy is the capacity and opportunity to make choices affecting one's welfare and to determine for one's self just what is one's interest. Thus, knowing that someone chooses to die, while not decisive to a moral assessment of carrying through the choice, is nonetheless a vital component.[22]

Beyond satisfying ourselves that someone has genuinely chosen death, we must ask whether the reasons for such a choice are compelling. This is a much more difficult and open-ended question, as there are very many different views about what could constitute compelling reasons for choosing death.

This sketch of what questions need to be asked when a death labeled suicide is to be morally assessed does not take us very far. All the really difficult work remains to be done. But that is just the point: there are no shortcuts to doing the difficult moral evaluations of choices for death provided by such labels as "suicide" or, one might add, "euthanasia." In the remainder of this book, we shall be examining just such principles and guidelines as might be used for assessing problematic choices for death. Further, we shall seek to apply these principles and guidelines to several especially complex cases.

Interlude: Observations on Historical and Contemporary Attitudes Toward Suicide

To many an ear this first question, "Does the person choose to die?" will be very strange. But to many others it will be far less strange than if asked even only ten or twenty years ago. The reasons for this are many, and herald a significant cultural change from the days in which suicide was automatically and vehemently condemned as sinful, unlawful, and morally heinous. A large part of that historical shift began in the last century with the perception that there were forces beyond the control of the will of individual agents that led to suicide. Soon this perception took the form of claiming that those who suicided were "mentally ill" and therefore beyond the bounds of moral responsibility. It thus became inappropriate to blame would-be suiciders for doing what was beyond their power to refrain from doing, and appropriate to regard them as persons in need of treatment for their illness. However exaggerated we have come to view this as a universal or scientific truth about suicide, it has two notable merits. The first is that it may, as a generalization about the greatest number of suicides, be true. This is worth remembering as we proceed to ask questions about the morality of choices for death: that in the most statistically frequent number of those choices, moral agency is at least severely diminished by forces not of the agent's choosing or doing. Consequently, moral blame (or praise) for suicide must be greatly qualified.

The second great merit of a scientific understanding of suicide, as it came increasingly to supplant a religious and moralistic view, is that it fostered real progress in human relations and an improvement in how formerly despised members of society were regarded. Treatment, rather than punishment, and understanding and sympathy, rather than condemnation, are real moral progress. Even priests, disposed by religious dogmas to refuse burial in consecrated ground to suicides, came increasingly to understand that moral blame was frequently inappropriate and consequently found ways to treat those who attempted suicide, successful suicides, and the survivors left behind with greater compassion and respect.

It might be thought that this was a sufficiently wide swing of the pendulum of social attitudes toward suicide as not to leave any ground uncovered. Yet in the movement from universal condemnation and barbaric treatment of suicide to the scientific detachment that understands suicide as caused and not chosen and its "victims" as in need of treatment rather than punishment, something of great significance did disappear: respect for the moral agency of those drawn to suicide. One way in which this lack of respect has been typicaly manifested in the view that suicide is a sickness has been the highly coercive and manipulative treatment in mental hospitals of those who attempt suicide. Some correction of our attitudes was therefore desirable, and perhaps inevitable.

But instead of finding the pendulum of public attitudes toward suicide seeking some greater balance in the center between blaming and excusing suicide, it seems now to be veering ninety degrees off in an entirely different direction. Instead of straight-out condemnations or pardonings of suicide, beyond even tolerance for a problematical practice, there is a growing tendency today to find suicide *praiseworthy*. This is reflected in a whole genre of books and articles, advocating a "right to suicide" and sometimes more extreme forms of "euthanasia" and "assisted suicide."[23] It can be found in the social reformist efforts of such organizations as EXIT in Great Britain and the Hemlock Society in the United States, whose very names imply much about their ideologies. EXIT has gone so far as to assemble a "how-to" manual on suicide, with very explicit directions on sufficient quantities of which drugs will cause death, how to acquire such drugs and so on.

These sorts of advocacy and organizations, I hasten to add, go well beyond the much more modest, reflective, and sensitive efforts at reform pursued by the likes of the hospice movement or organizations such as Right to Die. The latter are likely to advocate a "right to die," understood in something like the manner explicated in chapter six. The more egregious advocates of suicide, however, are disposed not to see the tragic dimensions of death, but rather are enamored of the supposed virtue of so exercising control over one's fate that they view leaving the world via suicide as the ultimate expression of individuality, freedom, and self-determination. Accordingly, they promote not a right to die for the already dying, but a right possessed by everyone to choose death by suicide, whatever one's circumstances. In this, they are part of "the romanticization of death" examined in chapter one.

But while the pendulum of public attitudes may be seeking a different axis than that which swings between scientific excusing and categorical condemnation of suicide, it is far from clear which direction it will move in now. One possibility is, of course, this romanticization of death, in which suicide is not merely noble but perhaps even, in time, obligatory. If the pendulum moves this way, we can expect to see social policies moving toward the creation of the likes of the "Ethical Suicide Parlors" envisioned by Kurt Vonnegut, Jr. Here those weary of life, and those whose lives are no longer "useful" to themselves or to others in an overpopulated world, may check into a state-run facility that attempts to satisfy their every erotic fantasy while benignly allowing painless administration of lethal dosages of deadly drugs.[24]

On the other hand, on this other axis the pendulum might move toward a far more soundly reasoned notion of a "right to choose death" which does not see death benignly and preserves our sense of death as burdensome, even tragic, for both those who die and those left behind. On this view, it might be supposed, there are compelling reasons for allowing persons to choose death, and for requiring of others that they respect such choices, even, perhaps, to the point in some cases of assisting such choices. The social implications of this view may require less in the way of positive promotion of such choices and more by way of simply removing social stigmata and legal barriers to carrying out one's considered choice for death.

Underlying both these possible directions for the pendulum of public opinion to swing is a notion of a right to suicide. It is a serious and increasingly important notion, and however great our difficulties in understanding just what counts as suicide, one that warrants careful examination.

VIII

THE RIGHT TO CHOOSE DEATH

> It is quite obvious that there is nothing in the world to which every man has a more unassailable title than to his own life and person.
>
> Arthur Schopenhauer
> "On Suicide"

> Every man ought to make his life acceptable to others besides himself, but his death to himself alone. The best form of death is the one we like.
>
> Seneca
> *Letters From A Stoic*

The claim that each of us possesses a right to choose death, or to suicide, is a different and farther-reaching assertion of a right than the right to die considered in chapter six. The right to die is asserted in the context of someone's dying, where death is imminent and unavoidable. What is wanted is a specification of what rights a dying person has to exercise some measure of control over her or his dying. But with the assertion of "a right to choose death" or "a right to suicide," something far more radical is being claimed, namely, that one has a right to choose death even when not dying. Much more is at stake than control over the conditions of dying; what is at stake is nothing less than whether one has, as a matter of moral right and potentially legal privilege, sanction "to take arms against a sea of troubles, and by opposing end them" (Hamlet).

To adopt the point of view that individuals possess a right to choose death by self-inflicted means is a considerable change of perspective from still conventional attitudes. Among other things, it would shift the burden of moral criticism from those who attempt or succeed in suicide to those who would intervene to prevent such efforts. If there is a right to suicide, then interference with the exercise of that right is *prima facie* wrong, and always in need of justification. The exercise of one's rights is conversely *prima facie* right, and needs no justification until challenged.

Further, numerous alterations in law and social institutions would be required in order to recognize this right. Police, psychiatrists, hospitals of all sorts, insurance companies, crisis intervention centers, prisons, and the military would all be enormously affected. But if there is a good case for a right to suicide, then the changes in public attitudes leading to sweeping changes in law, public policy, and institutional structures would all be for the better.

Three rather different grounds might be advanced in support of the claim to a right to suicide. These are (1) that each person's life belongs to oneself alone and, like other property, may be disposed of as the owner pleases; (2) that making such choices is an exercise of autonomy by competent moral agents and that such choices require the same respect as any other choice made by such persons; or (3) that making such choices as for one's own death is among the fundamental human rights that should be recognized as belonging to every human being. The first two of these grounds for a right to suicide suppose that such a right is directly derivative from a fundamental human right—to property, or for freedom; the third claims that choosing death is itself as fundamental a human right as property or freedom, that it needs no derivation or qualification as a second-order right. There are both arguments for and difficulties with each of these foundations for a right to suicide.

Life as Property

On this view, each person is regarded as having a unique relationship to his or her own life, one that might be called "nontransferable ownership." Our lives are our property, and, while a kind of property that cannot be given over to another, they are, like other property, something over which we have the right of disposition. Eike-Henner Kluge formulates the argument that uses this notion to derive a right to suicide as follows:

> Each and every one of us stands in a peculiar and unique relationship to his life. Our life is our own in the way in which nothing else is. We could characterize this relationship by calling it, perhaps somewhat tendentiously, nontransferable ownership. But we do own it: that is the major point. And as with anything we own in the full-blooded sense of that term, we have the right to dispose of it as we please. In particular, we have the right to advance it, to ruin it, or even to dispose of it altogether. In short, we have the right to end it if we so please, to commit suicide. . . . Suicide, therefore, is our right simply in virtue of a much more general right: the right to do with our own property as we please.[1]

Objections to this way of grounding a right to suicide are legion, the most familiar no doubt being a direct challenge to the presumption that each of us owns our life. Rather, it is claimed, our lives are "owned" by God, who lends them to us, or by the state, to whom we owe primary allegiance. Various Judaic-Christian theologies have maintained the former; the latter goes back at least to Plato and Aristotle. Notice that this is a disagreement simply about property *rights* and not about property; that is, it does not challenge the notion that human life can intelligibly and properly be regarded as property.

A more radical objection is Kluge's, for he holds that the notion of "nontransferable ownership" is "logically incoherent":

> What we own—in any full-blooded sense of that term—we can disown, give away, sell, or otherwise dispose of so that it becames the property of someone else. We cannot do this with our lives. Therefore whatever the unique relationship this bears to us, it cannot be one of ownership. In an extended sense of the term, that of *identity* would be a better candidate.[2]

But it might be objected against Kluge that his claim is too strong, for he regards "property rights" as too extensive, too absolute. We do not have such unlimited rights as he seems to suppose to the treatment and disposition of even that property we clearly own. Community interest in historical preservation, aesthetics, usefulness, the needs of everyone, and other such considerations limit rights of use to private property. Hence, while problematical, "nontransferable ownership" need not be "logically incoherent." All property rights are subject to some legitimate restraints, and in the case of owning one's own life we might say this restraint is that the right is "nontransferable."

I think this is essentially correct, that Kluge concedes too much to the notion of "property rights." But I do not think that the best way to see the limits of property rights is by supposing that one restraint they suffer is that where the ownership of our very lives is concerned, this is a "nontransferable" right. Rather, the limits that legitimately exist to our rights to control property are much greater than the right we have to life. So limited are property rights, in fact, that they are not fundamental in anything like the way a right to life, to freedom, to live with dignity, and the like are fundamental. This means that property is not a sufficiently weighty notion to carry anything so significant as a right to suicide.

Moreover, there is something quite demeaning to persons in the view that the interest we have in our very lives is anything like the interest we have in property. A grandiose way of saying this is that property is simply not a concept of sufficient ontological status to encompass human life. A more modest way is to say that we diminish the significance and value of human beings when we reduce the regard each of us has for our life to that which we might have for our car, or TV, or shoes. The value of human life is greater than any concept of property can incorporate. It is one of the perversions of a culture so enamored of material possessions and "property rights" that we would even for a moment suppose that something elevating was being claimed for persons when it is said that each of us has a right to dispose of our life as we see fit because it is our property.

Suicide as a Right of Autonomy

"Autonomy" means many different things in ethics, perhaps especially in medical contexts. The range is vast, stretching from a capacity for deliberation and choice to a right to self-determination to a duty required of all who would be moral agents. It is a term derived from the Greek *autos* (self) and *nomos* (rule, or law) and first applied to self-governance in the Greek city-states. In a far more individualistic era than any envisioned by the Ancient Greeks, it has come to apply to individuals, and, in the sense relevant to supporting a right to suicide, autonomy is a catchword stressing the capacity and freedom of persons to be self-governing, that is, to deliberate, make choices, and freely pursue one's own vision of the good. Accordingly, the Principle of Autonomy enjoins all of us to respect the right of others to be autonomous.

The right to autonomy, or self-determination, is often taken to be "fundamental," meaning that it is neither capable of nor in need of being justified by appeal to still more basic moral principles. (Just how to justify any basic moral principle is at the heart of ethical theory.) But the rights of self-determination are not "absolute" in the sense that they are completely unlimited. The standard limitation on one's right to be self-determining is doing harm to others, especially harm in the form of impinging on their rights. But autonomy can also be limited by obligations one has, or by some impairment in one's capacity to deliberate and choose. These three limitations to one's right to pursue the good as one sees fit—the interests and rights of others, one's own moral obligations, and impaired capacity for informed and free choice—are especially important qualifications when considering a possible right to suicide.

A right to suicide can be regarded as derivative from the fundamental right of self-determination. For those persons who see it as in their best interest to die, who freely choose this and pursue it, respect is owed. That respect must be shown by the rest of us in the form of noninterference with their pursuit of what they have chosen. In showing such respect, we are but abiding by the fundamental obligation to respect the autonomous choices of others entailed by the Principle of Autonomy.

M. Pabst Battin objects that this way of grounding a right to choose death cannot be uniformly applied, is too easily defeated, and leaves too much undecided or undecidable.[3] Suicide, treated as an overrideable right, "may provide unequal treatment for individuals whose grounds for suicide are the same, but who differ in their surrounding circumstances or their relationships to others."[4] Further, a right to choose death so variously overrideable means that in practice almost no one will ever have such a right. So extensive are the grounds for defeating a claim that suiciding is a right that no one, except perhaps the most isolated hermit on earth, will be in a position to claim suicide as a right. Therefore, finally, all the really hard work remains to be done: spelling out precisely when one does or does not have a right to suicide, under what circumstances, with what consequences, how to weight the interests of others, the extent of one's obligations to others, the requirements for competency, and so forth. Only a very fully articulated theory of rights and extensive casuistry would be adequate to this task.

It is difficult to see these objections to grounding a right to suicide in autonomy as very telling. It is clear that death can be rationally and autonomously chosen, that it can be done without violating one's obligations and even with benefit to others. The cases of Anne Marleybone, Samson, and perhaps Marcellus show this much. With enough information, we might say the same of Leslie Tharp and Betty Blue. But even so, it might be objected, this is a very narrow range of potential suicides, covering only clearly altruistic cases and a few others where suffering is unbearable and the persons are relatively detached from other persons and ordinary obligations. What is more, it seems to place the burden of justification once again upon the suicider, and one of the things claiming a right to suicide was intended to do was free one of this burden.

But suicide is an act that does not occur in a vacuum, and it is ordinarily not without very serious and often devastating consequences for others. Even if it can be claimed as a right, it is not inappropriate that one be very careful to assure that exercising that right is the right thing to do. Having a right to do something provides us some entitlement to do it; it does not assure that doing it is right. It is appropriate to set very high standards of justification for exercising a right to suicide, given how often it is undertaken in an ill-considered manner, how frequently suiciders suffer diminished competence from mental illness, and how widespread and serious are the consequences for others.

It is therefore not surprising or misguided that all the really difficult work in justifying the exercise of the right to suicide remains even after acknowledging one's right to make such a choice. But one might, understandably, desire a foundation for the right to suicide that makes this task less uncertain and better defined. This is what Battin seeks to provide in claiming that the right to suicide is not derivative from a fundamental human right, but is itself a fundamental human right.

Suicide as a Fundamental Human Right

The right to choose death by suicide should be construed as a "fundamental human right," Battin says, on a level with such other fundamental rights as life, liberty, and freedom of assembly, speech, and worship.

So understood, the force of ordinary consequentialist arguments, so powerful when suicide was understood as merely a "liberty" right, is undercut. This is because, I suppose, the exercise of fundamental rights is definitive of human good, and it is generally the case that showing one's act
to be an expression of such a right is sufficient to justify it. The advantages of being able to regard choosing death as a fundamental human
right are very considerable, not the least of which is that numerous very
difficult moral choices in medicine would be greatly simplified. For, once
we know someone prefers death to continued life, whatever their reasons for such a choice, in whatever circumstances it is made, deference
to that preference is obligatory.

Battin's argument for regarding suicide as a fundamental right is
straightforward:

1. "Individuals have fundamental rights to do certain sorts of things
    just because doing those things tends to be constitutive of human dig-
    nity."
2. Suicide is constitutive of human dignity.
3. Therefore, "we have a right to suicide (if and when we do) *because* it is
    constitutive of human dignity."[5]

Battin provides a sophisticated, supplementary argument to show that
fundamental human rights are not, contrary to most views, equally distributed. It is precisely because such rights are rooted in dignity that they
are not equally distributed, and suicide demonstrates this as clearly as anything might. Only sometimes is suicide constitutive of human dignity,
and only then is it a matter of right. The best candidates for those types
of suicide that do reflect dignity are euthanatic suicide, where there is unbearable suffering, most often from a terminal condition, as in the case
of Betty Blue; self-sacrificial suicides, such as Anne Marleybone; and suicides of principle and social protests, such as the monks who immolated
themselves to protest the war against Viet Nam, or Bobby Sands, the
Irish Republican Army prisoner who starved himself to death protesting
British occupation of Northern Ireland. In these sorts of cases, "one
chooses death instead of further life, because further life would bring
with it a compromise of that dignity without which one cannot consent
to live."[6] In general, it will be suicides that are "nonviolent" (not necessarily in means, but as they are intended to affect others) that will be constitutive of human dignity, and not those that are intended to do harm to
others.[7]

The sticking point for many will be the claim that suicide is constitutive
of human dignity. Besides sorting out the categories listed above, for which
this is an entirely plausible supposition, Battin suggests that we have difficulty in seeing this because of our long association of suicide with sin or
with mental illness; because we are too familiar with suicide that is hostile
to others or occurs among isolated, lonely individuals, and so on. But these
are contingent, not necessary, features of suicide, and their prevalence

may even be greater because of the cultural taboos that have been so strong against suicide. She cites with approval speculation that in the future suicide might become a preferred way of death and a great advantage to those "afflicted by terminal illness or old age."[8]

I am very sympathetic with Battin's argument, and with what she is trying to achieve by it, which I take to be, in the broadest sense, greater respect for the personhood of those drawn to suicide. Her emphasis upon the importance, even centrality, of human dignity is one I share. I have argued at length the moral necessity of respecting and preserving the dignity of the dying (chapter six). Part of this argument acknowledged the moral right of the dying to make choices that would hasten death. Since dying is part of living, the same arguments apply to the living. And where a choice for death is genuinely an expression or enhancement of human dignity, I do think it must be strictly respected, even admired, sometimes assisted.

Skeptical Reservation:
Rights and Human Dignity

However, both the major and minor premises of Battin's argument might be challenged. With respect to the claim that all human rights rest on human dignity, it might be wondered if the notion of human dignity is not too slender a reed upon which to rest a whole theory of human rights. In saying this, I do not pretend to know what would be adequate to justify appeals to human rights. I share an increasing skepticism, found at least in the philosophical literature, about the possibility of adequately grounding any theory of fundamental human rights. For me, the best reason for defending and seeking application of a theory of human rights is that such notions have historically been, and continue to be, of immense value to oppressed people in their struggles for freedom and justice. If we are to take seriously Tarrou's advice, always to side with the victims, we will recognize that notions of human rights have a use value that surpasses philosophical efforts at justification.

I am inclined to think that a right to suicide and its justification are better expressed as follows. There is a right to choose death when, and only when, doing so is the expression or enhancement of a person's human dignity. Choosing death is most likely to be such an expression in those nonhostile choices for death labeled euthanatic, self-sacrificing, and protest. We have a right to make such choices as a function of our right to live with dignity. This right, in turn, as argued previously, derives from our fundamental right to live and a theory of justice that specifies the minimal conditions necessary for each of us to attain life with dignity.

On this view, the right to suicide is less basic than on Battin's view, but it is, I think, less problematically grounded. Only a right to life is fun-

damental; other rights require the development of a theory of justice to derive, and with such a theory, a right to choose death can be supported. Justifying a right to life, in light of our earlier analysis of life as good and
death as necessarily evil, seems to me easier than justifying a whole pano-
ply of fundamental rights. At the same time, complexity is reintroduced
when it is realized that now we need also a theory of justice to attain a
fuller understanding of human rights.

In sum, I think there is a right to kill oneself, but only when doing so
serves human dignity. I do not think such a right is, in the fullest sense,
"fundamental." I do think, however, it is very extensive, more so even
than such a right would be if it were simply a "liberty" right. Just how extensive is the right to choose death, when doing so is consistent with
human dignity, awaits consideration of a second reservation about
Battin's position: to what degree is the choice for death constitutive of
human dignity?

Skeptical Reservation:
Choosing Death and Human Dignity

Problematic as the major premise of Battin's argument is—whether we
can ground a whole theory of human rights on the concept of human
dignity—many will have more difficulty with the minor premise, the
claim that "suicide is constitutive of human dignity." As carefully as
Battin qualifies this bold claim, limiting it to the most plausible subset of
suicides and discounting our prejudice to accepting it, there are still
other grounds for doubt. Two of these are especially worth considering.
The first is the notion, considered in chapter one, that there is greater
human dignity in resisting death than in accepting it. The second is that
human dignity being relational, and not entirely individualistic, the implications for what kind of human community we will live in with a far
more permissive attitude to suicide need looking at.

In the whole history of humanity, few perhaps have had as compelling reason for ending their lives as the victims of Nazi persecution in
the Warsaw Ghetto or those confined in the concentration camps become death factories. Every manner of humiliation and indignity was
wrought upon men, women, and children, from starvation to slavery,
from nakedness, freezing, and suffocation to filth, crowding, and torture. Several million human beings were murdered. An unknown number preempted murder by killing themselves. Still others resisted both imposed and chosen death, rarely with success, but with determination.
The resistance best known to the world occurred within the Warsaw
Ghetto during the last several months of its existence.

Adam Czerniakow was president of the Jewish Council of the Warsaw
Ghetto from 1938 until his death the day after the deportation decree
was issued for the Ghetto in July 1942. During most of that time he strug-

gled valiantly to ameliorate the suffering of the Jews, negotiating with the Nazis for better conditions, food supplies, schools for the children, economic lifelines, and all else needed for survival. Increasingly intolerable demands were made upon him to cooperate with the oppressors lest conditions become still more grim, and he did cooperate, up to the point of selecting and mobilizing the Jews for deportation to death camps.

The last promise he was able to extract from the Nazis in exchange for cooperation was that the children would be spared. When this promise was violated, in July 1942, Czerniakow broke, and killed himself. Others in the rapidly depleting ranks of the Jewish community escalated their resistance, finally now through armed combat. Some escaped; others had their murders delayed.[9]

I do not for a moment suggest this story shows any fault or blameworthiness on the part of Adam Czerniakow for his suicide. No one dares judge this man harshly in the light of the suffering he must have endured. Yet if our measuring rod is human dignity, surely there is more to be said for the vigorous resistance mounted by those who rebelled against Nazi practices of arbitrary murder, transport to death camps, and death by starvation. In this rebellion is a profound humanity, a dignity—even, in the classical sense, a nobility—that passive capitulation to oppression misses.

It might be objected, however, that this sort of example gravely distorts the issue as it confronts or is likely to confront most of us. Our choice will not be between passive capitulation to raw evil and heroic resistance, but rather between the much more subtle and inexorable undermining of our dignity through the ravages of natural aging, disease, and decline and self-determined death. Further, it is the exacerbation of these natural processes by the successes of high technology medicine, capable of prolonging life beyond any measure of usefulness or value, that we may more likely wish to escape by choosing self-inflicted death.

Even so, there is more to be said for resistance to death and its attendant limitations than there is for surrender to the social realities of dying. Much that one suffers in aging, at least in America, has little to do with "natural processes" and much to do with social realities of attitudes, economics, political organization and priorities, the practice of medicine, and the culture generally. In a society frequently deemed "ageist" for its glorification of youth and glamour and its consequent view of the elderly as "burdensome" and best hidden away, the first-order rational response by the elderly to being so regarded is *not* suicide. One does not hear the Gray Panthers urging upon the elderly suicide as a way out of the indignities imposed upon them by society. Rather, Maggie Kuhn and her peers urge upon us social organization, political lobbying, and vigorous resistance to the inadequate medical and social programs that breed hardship and humiliation for the aged in a society too little concerned with its senior members.

But when all this is said and done, there are left still those terribly troublesome cases where neither oppression nor social deprivation are at the root of misery. A variety of nearly pure human suffering emerges and no amount of explanation or argument will gloss over the dismal face of unmasked death. No trait of character, no social reform, no miracle of medicine, will restore bodily integrity or mitigate declining power. Some dying while still living, and even some living while not dying, is too unbearable to endure for persons who cherish their dignity. For these persons, there is no virtue or merit in suffering further: only death will bring surcease, and only their choosing death and acting on that choice will be consistent with their dignity as human beings. It would be at least insensitive, perhaps even cruel, for those whose lives will continue to deny to such persons a right to end their lives.

It is not always, perhaps not even chiefly, human intentions, social inequity, or aggressive medicine that victimizes people; sometimes it is life itself, the very fates controlled by no will, subject to the control of no power, that afflicts us. Maybe this was so for Leslie Tharp; to some degree it was so for Betty Blue. In such extreme cases, resistance to unbearable suffering will of necessity take the form of rejecting life and choosing death. Those who have chosen death as the last desperate attempt to act with waning dignity will have no regrets, and will be released from an existence they must have regarded as worse than nonexistence. We who live on will lament our losses. There is little to glorify when such choices are made, still less to criticize.

There is only this irony to reflect upon: resisting death yet living with human dignity means that sometimes human beings will exercise their right to choose death.

Rights, Community, and Human Dignity

A final reservation one might have about acknowledging a fundamental human right to suicide is rooted in concerns about the nature of the community in which we will live where there exists respect and social support for the exercise of such a right. Battin herself has considered this at some length and has identified a number of dangers, chief of which are a multitude of socially sanctioned ways of manipulating and coercing others into suicide. For those with declining power and dependent upon others, it would not be difficult, she supposes, to manipulate the circumstances of their existence in ways that would make death by suicide seem the more dignified course. This might take little more than not changing the wet sheets of incontinent, bedridden clients in a nursing home. Such maneuvers, coupled with an ideology promoting one's seizing control of fate by choosing suicide, tolerance and even encouragement by others for such choices, and supportive social institutions (Ethical Suicide Parlors?), could lead to severe abuses of very vulnerable persons.[10]

Battin does not think these dangers inconsequential, but in the end is willing to risk them for the greater good of recognizing a fundamental human right and respecting the genuinely informed and sensitive choices for death that will be made by those not manipulated or coerced. I have no quarrel with this assessment, although I feel little comfort or competence to speculate on what the social consequences of changing attitudes toward suicide will be in the future. My reservation is less one of predicting dire consequences than it is about all the messages that might be communicated in the present to those contemplating suicide. That is, I wonder if in approving of suicide as a human right we might be communicating not so much respect for persons as indifference.

A community that values its members does not respond to their most extreme sufferings by suggesting that they would be better off dead—even if this is true. Rather, it is incumbent upon each of us to do all in our power to mitigate that suffering, in every way short of killing or encouraging self-killing. The very best part of the dominant religious traditions in Western societies has always been the insistence upon creating a community that minimizes injustice and suffering, but holds that where such creeps in it must be spread about and shared. Not all suffering is meaningful; no good will or can result from it. But all suffering can be shared in some fashion. Notions of abiding with others and suffering together seem a much more humane and dignified response to hardship than assurances that it is permissible, and even the exercise of a basic human right, to kill oneself. In such a society, our resources for ameliorating suffering would be invested in hospices and not in ethical suicide parlors.

The objection here is not a slippery slope argument that by recognizing a right to choose death we will eventually arrive at a much worse society for everyone. Rather, it is an objection to communicating to people, in a social context, that others believe the most adequate response to their suffering is that they die, even if by their own hand. This seems to be in principle the wrong message to give another, suffering human being. It would be far better that our concern be expressed as a willingness on our part to share the burden of suffering, however we might, short of promoting the desirability of death.

But it may be that this is really an objection to no more than others *initiating* consideration of death as the escape from unwanted life. Suppose one were only responding to such a proposal from someone who felt their life was not worth going on with? Should the response be sympathetic and supportive, because the other person is simply considering exercising her or his rights?

I don't see that the issues are any different in responding to another's consideration of choosing death than they are if we ourselves intitiate such consideration by promoting choices for death as a matter of right and the exercise of dignity. It is still the case that in the most fully human community it would be better to nurture hope for meaningful life and share the burden of making life worthwhile than it would be to encourage an option to take a shortcut through this struggle to death. In either case, we would be failing in our duty to sustain one another in times of crisis, and failing to create the conditions of social existence within which alone human life can be worthwhile.

Like the other reservations about regarding choices for death as a fundamental human right, this one is more cautionary than decisive. Human dignity may be a tenuous basis on which to found all human rights, but there is no denying that it is vitally important, somehow connected to any notion of rights, and a compelling consideration in assessing the propriety of any choice for death. Suicide may only sometimes be "constitutive" of human dignity, but in those cases in which it is, there is more than merely adequate reason to respect someone's choice to elect death by self-inflicted means. And now here, while acknowledging, even encouraging a right to choose death may not be the appropriate first (or even second) response of a decent community, there is no good reason to think it an improper response in the right circumstances and at the right time. Everything turns on filling in these specific details, for the limits of decision making on the basis of abstract principles are severe.

In another sense, the task is to find that balance between elevating individual choice to the point where community is rendered impossible, and denying persons the exercise of their rights because allowing such is regarded as not good for them or for others. With respect to suicide, it is surely desirable to eliminate the social stigma that presently attaches to nearly all suicide and move a great ways toward a more tolerant, even respectful understanding of what motivates those drawn to self-destruction in a wide variety of circumstances. But it cannot be desirable to move so far as to give open-ended permission, even encouragement, to persons in all or even very dire circumstances to exercise a right to die. A decent society finds ways of caring for those even in the most extreme distress; rarely is it the case that such caring is best done by encouraging death, through either suicide or euthanasia. Rarely, I said, but not never. For neither is it the case that in a decent society we would burden those for whom death is in their best interest with the sole responsibility for ending their lives, any more than we burden everyone with sole responsibility for sustaining their lives when this is best. Thus there might have been still more dignity in Betty Blue's choice to die had she been assisted, rather than left alone to drink Drano. Indeed, when individual responsibility for either sustaining life or choosing death is this severe, we do not have community at all.

In the final analysis, we do not serve the cause of ensuring human dignity by social mechanisms for making death easy and painless, by promoting self-inflicted and socially encouraged death for those whose ongoing lives are burdensome to themselves or others, any more than we respect

dignity when we go to great and repressive lengths to prevent all suicide and every other means of choosing death.

We need to guard against the illusions that prevent clear vision about
suicide as much as about other forms of death. It will not do to romanticize
suicide as a rational, desirable, rightful choice—even though it can be all
these things. It is worth reminding ourselves, with the novelist Joyce Carol
Oates, that by and large suicide is "a consequence of the employment of
false metaphors."

> It is a consequence of the atrophying of the creative imagination: the fail-
> ure of the imagination, not to be confused with gestures of freedom, or re-
> bellion, or originality, or transcendence. To so desperately confuse the
> terms of our finite contract as to invent a liberating Death when it is re-
> ally brute, inarticulate Deadness that awaits . . . .[11]

Conclusion

I believe people have a right to decide, for a vast variety of reasons
and in highly diverse circumstances, that their lives are not worth continuing. I believe further that they frequently have the right to act accordingly on such assessments and end life. Sometimes these decisions and actions are not simply an exercise of a right; they are the right decisions
and actions.

The right each of us has to choose death is a right bred both by the entitlement to liberty each possesses as an autonomous person deserving
moral respect and, still more fundamentally, by the requirements of
human dignity itself. Not much suicide is an expression or enhancement
of human dignity, but that which is occurs as a matter of human right, a
right derived from considerations of justice and our fundamental right to
live with dignity.

Recognition of such a right raises very difficult questions about the
proper response of other members of a community to the exercise of the
right. The first obligation would seem to be to shed whatever moralistic
prejudices we retain about the wrongness of suicide. The second is not
thereby to approve all suicide and set about making those changes in
law, medicine, and social institutions required to facilitate suicide.
Rather, I have argued, the better course is to evaluate carefully each would-
be suicide's ostensible desire for death to see if it is genuine and supported by compelling reasons.

Even after this is done, however, there is much more that a decent community would do to try to share its concerns and resources with those persons wanting to leave it forever. These range from suicide prevention centers (whose powers do not exceed the limits of respecting the freedom
and dignity of competent persons), to imaginative ways of relieving
another's suffering through sharing, to hospices. As with those drawn

to suicide, for whatever reasons in whatever circumstances, those who live on must seek to expand stultified imagination in finding modes of caring sufficient to deter a choice for death. Only as a last resort, after all other forms of caring have failed, does respect for another's right to choose death obligate us not to interfere, and sometimes to assist. These last are the most difficult cases of all, and the sort we shall consider next.

IX

THE LIMITS OF PERSONAL AUTONOMY

THE CASE OF

DONALD/DAX COWART

> I was a hostage to the current state of medical technology.
>
> Dax Cowart, 1984

> [Mr. Cowart] is confused, not so much about whether he wants to die, but about whether others want him to die.
>
> Robert Burt
> *Taking Care of Strangers*

At the age of 26 Donald Cowart was nearly immolated in an explosion and ensuing fire that destroyed his father and left Donald critically injured. The Cowarts were inspecting a piece of Texas real estate, Donald having just joined his father in the real estate business. Unknown to them, a propane gas main had been leaking for several days and had accumulated a substantial pool of gas in a dry creek bed. When the Cowarts were ready to leave, attempts to start their car ignited this pocket of gas, killing the senior Cowart in a very few moments, and propelling Donald, in flames, down a half-mile run on the road. There he collapsed and was found by a local farmer who had come to investigate the explosion and fire. Donald first asked that help be summoned for his father. Then he asked the farmer for a gun, that he might kill himself. The man called for an ambulance, but as to Donald's request for a gun, he said, "I can't do that."[1]

Those were words Donald Cowart was to hear frequently for more than a year, most often in response to some request from him for relief of his intense suffering or for surcease of life-prolonging treatments. These were sometimes the same. Donald Cowart was first taken to a small community hospital—after asking the ambulance driver not to take him to any hospital—where, over his continued protests to any treatment, he was stabilized and transferred to a major medical center in Dallas. He was found to be suffering deep burns, in excess of 65 percent total body burn, second and third degree. By July 1973, when Donald's accident occurred, enormous progress had been made in the treatment of serious burns. For better or worse, Donald Cowart was to be the recipient of these medical and technological advances.

When Donald first presented to the emergency room of a hospital, there was little attention paid to his professed desires. He was in an immediately life-threatening situation, and all concern was understandably directed towards saving his life. Thus his requests—to the farmer, that he be given a gun, to the ambulance driver, that he not be taken to the hospital, to the ER team, that he not be treated—were all ignored. What is more difficult to understand is how Donald Cowart remained so adamant in his profession of this desire and how uncomprehending and unaccommodating his caregivers were of such requests all during the many long months he endured treatment.

Treatment consisted of innumerable surgeries: skin grafts for his burns; to remove an infected eye; to attempt (unsuccessfully) to restore vision in his remaining eye; to amputate nearly all the fingers on both hands; to repair (again unsuccessfully) the elbow joint of his right arm; to implant prosthetic eyes, and so on. Far the worst of the treatments were the daily Hubbard tankings. These consisted of Donald's being immersed in a large tank of water, laced with Clorox, to cleanse his many open sores. During these tankings his dressings would be peeled off, and afterwards new dressings applied. These baths were excruciatingly painful, the more so because of the Clorox in the water, the powerfully air conditioned room in which they were administered, the minor sedation administered beforehand, the mechanical and seemingly unfeeling application of dressings by technicians, the raucous music replete with commercials for cosmetics that blared throughout, the fact that they occurred every day, and the fact that they were administered at the convenience and direction of the hospital and its staff and employees whatever Mr. Cowart's protests. For all this, they were an essential component of Donald Cowart's treatment, for without such cleansings, massive sepsis would overwhelm and destroy him.

Donald was not impressed with the treatments, not grateful to have had his life saved, not desirous of continuing this regimen at all. He repeatedly protested, sought release, attempted to persuade friends and caregivers to help him die, and finally attempted to engage a lawyer to get him released from the hospital that he might go home to die. No one, it seems, was very sympathetic with his requests; at least no one—no friend, relative, nurse, physician, or lawyer—cooperated with Donald's requests. This would have been readily understandable, perhaps, had Donald been in continuous shock, or mentally unbalanced, or making morally outrageous demands. But none of these was the case, although clearly some of his physicians tried to demonstrate that he was not mentally competent to make his own choices and did regard those choices as altogether morally unacceptable.

It would be easy to view Donald Cowart, prior to his devastating accident at least, as an "American type." The type is that of the "rugged individualist," if not peculiar to, at least prevalent in the American West. He was a man who took great pride in his independence and self- reliance. Donald was an exceptionally handsome and athletic young man. In high school he distinguished himself as a running back on the football team. After high school and college, he became a pilot in the Air Force and flew a number of missions in Viet Nam. Back home in Texas he rode broncos bareback in the rodeo and considered a career as a commercial airline pilot while working with his father, with whom he was very close. He describes himself as having always been "willful" and "stubborn," and those who knew him early, and those who have come to know him since his tragic accident, would likely agree with this self-characterization.

Another dimension of Donald Cowart, consistent with his culture and character, stable throughout his life, is his commitment to "libertarian" principles of political philosophy. Donald Cowart has always believed, it would seem, in the supremacy of the individual, in the unfettered right to personal freedom and self-determination except where the exercise of such freedom unreasonably interferes with the rights of others. It was thus for him the more incredible, and outrageous, that throughout his prolonged hospitalization, numerous surgeries, and long rehabilitative therapies so little consideration was accorded his wishes, desires, and attempts at decision making. How did this occur? How might it be thought justified?

Far from being "mentally unbalanced," Donald Cowart was remark- ably lucid and articulate throughout some of the most difficult times of his extended treatment. After nearly a year of enduring unwanted surgeries and tankings, Donald was more adamant than ever that he wished to be released and go home, knowing full well that he could not survive long if he did so. Dr. Robert White, a consulting psychiatrist, was called upon to examine Donald. White found the case so extra- ordinary that he made a 30-minute videotape of an interview with Donald Cowart which he intended to use for clinical teaching purposes. It is initially through this tape that Cowart's case came to the attention of a far larger audience.

A Videotape

The tape, titled "Please Let Me Die," is a graphic depiction of Donald Cowart's mental and physical condition. The camera work especially is very intrusive, emphasizing the degree of maiming and disability suffered by Donald. It begins with one of the daily Hubbard tankings to combat infection in Cowart's open sores. He does not speak, nor does anyone speak to him. Instead, he is lifted onto a pallet, which is then connected to chains from an overhead lift. He is raised, moved over the tank, and lowered into it. While there is no speaking, there is plenty of sound, ranging from the chilling clanking of the chains against the metal tub, to Cowart's soft moans, to the harsh blaring of a radio listened to by the therapists. The camera then cuts to Donald Cowart's room where we find Dr. White, sitting beside the bed, interviewing him. It is while they speak, calmly, deliberately, with feeling and conviction, always with restraint and rationality, that the camera offers the visual counterpoint of the grotesque. We see that Donald Cowart has only stumps for hands, what remains of his fingers at this point—prior to amputation—having been encased in a fold of skin. We observe the moonscape of his skin, that he cannot bend his arms, that his pencil-thin legs can hardly be moved, that his once handsome face is now largely featureless, lacking eyes, ears, most of his nose, and with Vaselined lips encasing his mouth. At one point we are shown photos of an earlier Donald Cowart, plunging through the line to gain yardage as a football running back, standing next to a fighter plane, riding a bronco bareback in a rodeo.

The tape is not yet over. It does not end until we have returned to the tank room, where Donald is being raised now from the chemical bath to be dried and have fresh dressings applied. The full horror of his situation is inescapable, as now, with every nerve ending in his body worn raw, he cries out in pain at every careful and careless touch. The impression of a life destroyed beyond all redemption is powerfully conveyed.

When viewing this tape, one needs no expertise in psychiatry to discern the evident clarity and deep conviction of Donald Cowart's words. His mind is lucid and he is most articulate, as when, in this part of the conversation, he insists upon a patient's right to determine the course of treatment:

> What really . . . astounds me . . . is that in a country like this where freedom has been stressed so much and civil liberties, especially during the last few years, how a person can be made to stay under a doctor's care and be subjected to the painful treatment such as the tankings which are very painful, against this person's wishes, especially if he has demonstrated the ability to reason . . . The way I see it, who is a doctor to decide if a person lives or dies?

There would seem to be two things impelling Donald Cowart to prefer death to continued life. The first, obviously, has to do with the incredibly difficult conditions of his present existence. He is surely grieving the loss of his father, with whom he was close; his powerlessness has undermined his sense of independence and self-reliance, is new and very frustrating, and appears not even to be of concern to others; and he is in continuous, unimaginable pain. By itself, this would suffice to undermine the will to live of even the strongest person. But on top of this lies another burden: Donald Cowart sees nothing in the future that persuades him to endure the present, not even the slim hope of a future worth living for or in.

> All my life I have been active in sports. I have played golf, surfed and rodeo . . . I've played football, basketball in school, run track and I've been very oriented to athletics in general. And now, I think, at best, I could just be rehabilitated to the extent where I could make it alone rather than be able to do things I really enjoy. If I were to enjoy myself after being rehabilitated, I think it would have to be by changing completely the things I am interested in. I don't think that this is very likely, that I would become interested in other things as I have been before . . . . [T]here's no way I want to go on as a blind and a cripple.

Robert White found Donald Cowart to be rational and competent. He could not, therefore, satisfy the wish of at least some of Cowart's physicians that Cowart be declared mentally ill so that state civil commitment laws could be invoked and treatment forced upon him against his will. Nonetheless, White was no more eager than any of the myriad of other health professionals who had dealt with Cowart to see him die. Perhaps this was especially poignant for Robert White, as he, uniquely, knew both how salvageable Donald Cowart's life was and how deeply and seriously Donald felt about wanting out. White had listened carefully and respectfully to Donald. He seems to have convinced Donald to continue talking with him, and after several weeks of doing so, to go on with treatment. It is not clear that Cowart had a change of heart or mind about wanting to live; it is clear, however, that as soon as someone took him seriously, listened carefully, treated his professions respectfully, he seemed more willing to cooperate with what were represented to him as medical imperatives.

One argument that may have carried some weight was that by enduring more treatment and rehabilitative therapy he would be in a better position to end his own life, if he still so desired, and would not need to depend upon or impose upon others to help him do so. It was one of Cowart's surgeons, speaking in a documentary film made about the case, who used this argument on him and believed it to be efficacious. Cowart's account is somewhat different. His recollection is that he consented to further surgery in order to assure an earlier release from the hospital. Even here, however, he believes he was misled and manipulated. He was told, by a nurse in this instance, that whether or not he had further skin grafts he would recover, and the only issue was whether it would be sooner or later. Presumably the surgery would mean an earlier release. Later Donald learned that this was not so, that without this surgery he would likely have died of gangrene. Again, when he consented to surgery to amputate his fingers "at the first joint," he believed this meant he would lose the outermost digit of each finger. Only afterward did he learn that surgeons counted joints from the hand outward, not from the fingertips inward.

After fourteen months, Donald was released from hospital, his wounds sufficiently healed to enable him to live on his own. There were still many months of painful therapy ahead, during which he needed to learn to walk again and to function now as a blind man. For a while he lived with his mother, but there was too much conflict between them for this to be satisfactory to either. Later he lived in his own house, with a couple of friends. Throughout he struggled with the question of whether life was worth going on. He entertained frequent thoughts of suicide, and at least twice attempted suicide. One night, while still living with his mother, he walked out to the highway and stood on the edge of the road listening to and feeling the trucks roar by. He considered lying down on the road. Later he attempted to slash a wrist, gripping a razor with his one working digit, his left thumb. Still later he attempted to overdose on tranquilizers and sleeping pills. Throughout he suffered from serious sleep disorders, continued pain, and despair about the conditions of his life.

Donald Cowart did not die, but "Donald" did. He changed his name to "Dax" and went on to develop those other sorts of interests and activities that once held little appeal. He has, by his own account, become "more cerebral." The change of name heralds more than a change of self-concept; for Donald/Dax Cowart it would seem accurately to reflect a real change of essential self.

In recent years, Dax Cowart has married, divorced, gone to and completed law school. He has also appeared at public gatherings with some frequency—at seminars for medical students, at workshops organized by Concern for Dying, at medical ethics conferences for health professionals. He has become a forceful, informed, and highly articulate advocate of patient rights. Dax Cowart says he is glad to be alive, but he continues to believe that he and all others have a moral right to decide whether to accept life-prolonging medical treatment, that no one else has this right, and that especially no one has the right to force upon unwilling others their conception of what is good, right, or dutiful for that other person. While he remains angry about the many abuses of rights he suffered, he is clearly not bitter. He hopes in time to practice personal injury law, that he may represent others whose rights are in jeopardy. Most of all, he says, he would like to ensure that no one ever again suffers the imposition of undesired medical treatment, however beneficial others believe such treatment to be.

The Case for No Treatment

The case for not treating a patient like Dax Cowart, even when doing so is the only way to prolong the life of someone not terminally ill, is powerful. The case made by someone with the courage, experience, intelligence, and sincerity of Dax Cowart himself is compelling. The argument has largely been made in the recounting of Dax's history and his opinions about how he should have been treated. It consists essentially of two sorts of claims, which might be summarized as follows:

1. It should be the absolute right of competent persons to decide whether to undergo or continue to undergo medical treatment. Respect for the autonomy of a human being requires that others accede to that person's choices when no other person's vital, essential interests are at stake. Dax clearly demonstrated that he was autonomous in all relevant respects, and no one else could or did have a a greater interest in his life. Hence his values and choices alone should govern treatment decisions.

2. No worthwhile social good results from the imposition of an unwanted "good" upon another against his or her will. In forcing life-prolonging treatment upon an unwilling patient, medicine (and society generally) does not affirm its commitment to "the value of human life," as might be claimed. Rather, what happens is that respect for freedom and self-determination is diminished, and human dignity is undermined.

More might be said. For example, on the basis of the immediately preceding claims, a thorough critique of the arrogance that underlies much of medical paternalism might be launched. Further, the willingness to impose such abstract principles as "the value of human life" upon others, especially others who are vulnerable, relatively powerless, and suffering greatly, does not imply moral sensitivity but rather just its opposite. But these are familar enough claims in today's climate, and need not be belabored. And there is, after all, an argument to be made in favor of treating Dax Cowart, however much he protests.

The Case for Treatment:
The Value of Life

That argument might proceed on two levels. The first is to dispute the values invoked by Dax Cowart; the second is to disagree about the facts on which judgments are allegedly based. Consider first disputes about values. A direct challenge might be launched against Cowart's invocation of such a minimally qualified right of autonomy. While it is conceded that Cowart is, in all relevant respects, acting autonomously, it can be argued that respect for even fully autonomous choices is not the most important consideration. More important still is what one chooses and whether it is defensible on some morally substantial ground other than (merely) that one has autonomously chosen it. By this more sturdy test, it might be suggested, Cowart's choice to reject life-prolonging treatments and die is not one that should be respected.

What, then, are these "more sturdy" and "substantial" values that Cowart is thought wrongly to ignore? There are three plausible candidates, falling under the general rubrics of the value of life, obligations to specific others, and community welfare.[2] The first of these is the familar view that nothing is so valuable as life itself, and that any action that would shorten or terminate life is wrong at least insofar as it destroys something of intrinsic or even absolute value. However great Cowart's suffering, it does not justify his choosing to destroy that which has incomparable value, his very life.

Views on the "value of life" were explored in chapter two, where it was conceded that death was, for every person and on each occurrence, an evil. Yet I also argued there that while this was so, it did not follow that death was the greatest evil one might suffer; neither, therefore, would preferring death to the continuation of certain forms of life be to choose a lesser value. Given the severity and the intensity of Donald Cowart's suffering, coupled with his genuinely dim prospects for a satisfying future, he cannot be reasonably faulted for thinking that it would be worse for him to go on living than to die. This evaluation has every mark of being a rational and reasonable one.

Further, it could be said that Donald Cowart's choice for death is not a denial of the value of life, but is rather an affirmation of the importance of life as lived being of a sufficient quality that the person whose life it is values it. The forcible, unwanted prolongation of a life found to be without value by the person whose life it is is as much an assault on that person's dignity as is the forcible, unwanted termination of his or her life. It is thus a mistake to say that anything Mr. Cowart attempted to choose constituted a denial of the value of life; on the contrary, it is more likely that he has a far more sensitive appreciation of life's value and its tragic possibilities than the critic who doggedly and unqualifiedly asserts the absolute value of human life.

The Case for Treatment:
Duties to Others

A second, potentially stronger, objection to Mr. Cowart's choice for death is that in pursuing such a choice, he fails to discharge specific obligations to others, or in some other fashion imposes upon them undue harm.³ This is a very serious matter, for everyone's rights to choose and act are constrained by the harm that may be done others and by the obligations they have incurred to others. But the notion that one's obligations to others might extend so far as to require one to go on living—or even to make every effort to go on living—whatever the cost to oneself, is a peculiar one, and was examined earlier. Nonetheless, it is worth raising again in the specific case of Dax Cowart, and asking who would be harmed and what Dax might owe to such persons.

Surely Dax's friends and family will be hurt by his death, most especially his mother. It is she, as next of kin, whom Dax's doctors have turned to for permission to treat him, and it is she who has suffered already the loss of her husband and fears for her son's life. There is no question that she will suffer with his death, perhaps even more than she already does abiding with him through this long and grueling course of treatment. But those who love Dax Cowart will suffer no matter whether he endures more treatment or dies, and the question is not really one of what course will lead to the least suffering for others, but which actions by Dax they have a right to expect he will take. Whatever their interest in his continuing to live, have they the right to demand of Dax that he do that which will be best for them, but which, according to his own thoughtful consideration, he believes will be less good for him? It is not sufficient that others, in making claims upon Dax, merely show that one course of action by him will be less painful for them than another course of action. What they must further demonstrate is that Dax *owes* it to them to act as they prefer, that in virtue of some incurred or assumed or natural obligation by him he must do what is best for them at whatever expense to himself.

Difficult as this may be to show, it is surely not in all cases impossible. After all, people can take on obligations under which they are in duty bound to sacrifice their very lives, so it is not inconceivable at all that one might be obligated to go on living for the benefit of others. A classic, if trivial, example of the latter would be that of an airplane pilot overwhelmed with the pointlessness of life and sorely tempted to suicide being at least obligated not to do so at 35,000 feet with a planeload of passengers. But we do not really need here—or in very many other places—an abstract argument purporting to prove the nature and limits of anyone's obligations. It should prove adequate, to a reasonable consideration of this case and others like it, to assess the balance of goods and harms, or benefits and burdens, to all parties in conflict.

The first thing to note in this regard is that while others may suffer increased grief with Dax's demise, none is at risk of losing his or her own life or even some essential support to sustaining life. That is to say, in effect, that no one has as much at stake as Dax himself in whether he continues to live, and the decision on whether to continue to live would thus seem, on this ground, most appropriately to be his.

Moreover, against the harm others may suffer by Dax's death is the burden to be borne by Dax in continuing to live. As is evident, this is a heavy burden, the more so for being so complex. There is in the first place the intense and prolonged suffering of his injuries and treatments. The pain these engender may be so compelling, so overwhelming, that other harms seem insignificant. They are nonetheless real, and need to be noted. There is, for instance, the very real loss of the future. Even if Dax lives, what might have been for him now cannot be: his body is radically altered, the kinds of experiences and relationships available to him will be very different, his interests and activities will of necessity be different, and his opportunities for a wide variety of experiences have been reduced.

All of these only hint at what, should Dax endure the present pain and go on living, may prove to be as great a burden: the construction of a new self. Perceptively, Dax was well aware of this burden, as when he said, "If I were to enjoy myself after being rehabilitated, I think it would have to be by changing completely the things I am interested in. I don't think that this is very likely. . . ." The question here is not whether such a transformation of self is possible—indeed, we know in retrospect that it is, because to a very large degree it has been accomplished—but whether it is fair or just to impose upon Dax Cowart the expectation, or even more, the *duty*, of making such changes.

Again, in the abstract, it may be quite all right to expect someone to radically transform himself or herself. Suppose a woman has a long history of chopping up others with an ax; then quite understandably we might wish she would change herself considerably and we might express this as something she ought to do or is obligated to do for the benefit of the rest of us. Dax Cowart is neither an abstraction nor an ax murderer. He is rather the victim, first, of a tragic accident, and second, of imposed and undesired medical treatment. He is (or was) a person of whom no sufficently serious moral criticism could be leveled that would warrant the claim that he ought, really, to have worked to become a very different sort of person.

An argument could be made that it is in Dax's *interest* to work at developing new interests, activities, and hobbies, at least if he is to go on living. And that is surely true. But it is quite another matter to make the very much stronger claim that he must do so, that doing so is some sort of obligation owed others. That claim is far too strong, and unfair. Dax Cowart, surely, owes it to no one to become something other than the (good) person he already was. If he *chooses* to endure the hardships of becoming still another sort of person, we can have nothing but admiration for his courage and determination. Such a choice would be heroic, but never obligatory.

There is another group of persons for whom it might be thought that Dax Cowart is obligated to continue treatment. These are, in the strict sense, neither friends nor family, but rather the health professionals who are treating him. At least one such person, Dr. Baxter, who directed much of the care rendered Dax, believed Dax was obligated to accept treatment in part because it was his, Baxter's, duty as a physician to deliver it. Moreover, Baxter regarded Dax Cowart's demands for the cessation of treatment as designed to "manipulate" others.[4]

It is tempting to explain such views—such a seeming parody of reasoning—in terms of the arrogance of one so persuaded of the right-eousness of his work and ordinarily unchallenged in the exercise of his power that he does not see how fundamentally disrespectful and oppres-sive such attitudes can be to patients. Whatever the merits of such an explanation of Baxter's attitudes, it will not suffice. It would be better to see if some fuller account of such views can be offered, and then test the grounds on which they might be thought justified.

The values and reasoning behind Baxter's views might be of the following sort:

1. The main obligation of a physician is to deliver good medical care.

2. The greatest good that can be achieved through providing good medical care is the saving of human lives.

3. Dax Cowart is a patient capable of deriving the greatest benefit from good medical care because it can save his life. For him willfully to reject this benefit is equivalent to choosing suicide and, what is more, making his caregivers complicit in doing so.

4. For Cowart to forsake life-sustaining treatment, then, is wrong, for three reasons:
   a. it amounts to choosing suicide, which is intrinsically wrong;
   b. it makes physicians complicit in an act which is intrinsically wrong and which violates their role obligations as physicians;
   c. it prevents physicians from doing that which they ought to do, *viz.*, deliver good medical care and, most of all, save life.

5. Therefore, it is wrong for physicians not to treat Cowart, and wrong for him to ask that they not treat him.

"Good Medical Care"

Let us consider each of these claims in turn. It would be difficult to find anyone who would disagree with so general a claim—almost a truism—that a physician's first obligation is to deliver good medical care. Of course everything turns upon the understanding of "good medical care." For those who advance an argument of the sort under consid-eration, good medical care must be understood as that which heals injury and illness, promotes health, and generally prolongs life. Hence the corollary view, 2 above, that the greatest good a physician can do is to save life.

There are certainly other views of what counts as good medical care and of the obligations of physicians. One alternative view would place the emphasis upon a physician's obligation first to provide good *patient* care, without presuming that in all cases this means healing or prolonging life. After all, not all injuries or illnesses can be cured, health cannot always be restored, and certainly life is not always extendable. Moreover, these are not, for all persons, in all conditions and at all times, necessarily good things to seek. The vulnerable and the ill—all of us at times—still need to be cared for even if we cannot be cured, restored to health, or enabled to live longer. It is certainly a proper function—perhaps the first obligation—of those who would be healers to care for their patients and seek to do what is best for a patient, even where this may, in the extreme case, mean helping one to die sooner rather than to live longer. How far physicians may go in helping terminally ill patients to die is hotly disputed, but none, surely, deny the duty to provide comfort and concern.

In any case, the point is that it is quite possible to understand by "good medical care" placing an emphasis more upon catering to patients' self-determined choices of best interest than upon a physician's exercise of technical skills. By doing so, one gets a very different view of patient benefit and of a physician's duties.

Knowing and Doing the Best
for a Person

The rejoinder to these caveats on the first two premises is implicit in the third. That response would go like this: Dax Cowart is not terminally ill, and need not be. His life is salvageable, and although he cannot be restored to the full level of functioning he enjoyed before his terrible accident, he can go on to lead an altogether meaningful and potentially satisfying life. Physicians do their patients no good, on either account of how physicians ought to do good, by acceding to a patient's ill-considered or misinformed desires. In the midst of his suffering, Dax Cowart cannot adequately assess his future prospects. Health professionals with clinical experience of patients in similar plights and with medical expertise about what is possible in the way of restoring bodily functioning are better situated to evaluate such prospects. Possessed of such expertise, they properly have the determining say in what treatments are indicated.

There is nothing new in this rejoinder, and there is some truth in it. Experienced clinicians know first of all about how bodies function, and to some degree they know the prognosis on how a particular body is capable of functioning in the future. Good clinicians do acquire a kind of wisdom about the dynamics of a person's response to illness and injury. This can give insight both into how an injured person feels at the moment, at a certain stage of disability, and into how that person is likely to feel later, after a measure of improved bodily functioning. Such expertise as this is at the very core of clinical medicine. It constitutes a body of knowledge essential to the practice of good medicine, good nursing, and good patient care generally. And yet for all that, the acquisition of such expertise falls short of conferring upon its acolytes an entitlement to function as moral decision-makers for others.

The fallacy here is one that Robert Veatch has aptly termed "the generalization of expertise."[5] It consists of presuming that technical proficiency confers upon its holders special moral competency, the ability to choose the morally correct course in a situation in which values are in dispute. Beyond possessing this special competency, it is also supposed that those with expertise in how things work have thereby the right to exercise decision-making authority in situations where there is disagreement about what ought to be done.

Both these presumptions are in need of justification, and neither is obviously true. Indeed, there is compelling reason to think that having expert knowledge in how things work and what can be done is not always the best preparation for deciding what ought to be done, not only in medicine, but in matters of public policy—for instance, the development and deployment of nuclear weapons. Technicians have frequently not proven to be the wisest policy makers, blinded as they sometimes are by what is possible, and failing to question whether being able to do something is sufficient warrant for supposing it desirable to do.

Moreover, even if we did grant that those who knew best what was the case also knew best what ought to be the case, it still would not follow that they ought to be the ones to choose. Distinct from the "substantive" question of what ought to be done is the "procedural" one of who ought to decide what to do. (This is, of course, a frequently misleading distinction, at least in that it is sometimes the case that only through following the correct procedure is it possible to arrive at the substantively correct decision. Such at least is the fundamental faith underlying democracy.) Merely knowing what would be best to do does not confer upon one the right to choose to do it, as every parent who struggles to maintain a cordial relationship with an adolescent knows only too painfully. Often it is more important that the right person make a choice than that the right choice be made.

Thus, to return to Dax Cowart's case, it is not necessarily true that even very competent clinicians know what (morally) ought to be done in his case or know what is best for Dax himself, or even if they do know these things, it is not necessarily true that they have the right to implement their view of what is good, right, and true. To act on their beliefs and values in Dax's case would be (was) a very heavy-handed paternalism, overriding the clearly expressed preferences of a clearly competent patient. Such strong paternalism carries with it a heavy burden of justification. On very few accounts of what justifies paternalism could this burden be met in the present case.

Thus the argument that holds that Dax Cowart ought to accept treatment for his burns and that physicians would be wrong to do other than aggressively treat him begs the question at a number of crucial points. In particular, it unjustifiably assumes that (A) physicians know better than Cowart what is right to do or best for him; (B) they, not he, have the right to determine which treatments he should undergo; (C) clinicians are obligated to deliver treatment, in this case even to an unwilling and resisting patient. Worse than merely begging the question, these assumptions are, on any careful examination, largely unsupportable. It is gratuitous to suppose that refusing to undergo life-prolonging treatment is equatable with suicide, and a mistake to regard suicide as "inherently wrong" in any case. These errors, along with disputable notions of a physician's role obligations, render the conclusion that Dax Cowart's physicians must deliver life-prolonging treatment and that he must cooperate vacuous.

My own view, as I indicated above, is that a properly formulated version of A, that experienced clinicians often know what is best for patients, is true. But the generalization of B, that the acquisition of such knowledge confers upon clinicians the sole right to make treatment decisions, is false, and specifically, as applied to Dax Cowart, is both false and morally wrong. Finally, I believe, as already indicated, that C, the notion that physicians are obligated to deliver life-sustaining care even in opposition to the wishes of competent patients is very wrong, an undue burden on clinicians and usually disrespectful and not beneficial to patients.

Disputes about the Facts

We have thus far proceeded as if we knew quite clearly what the relevant facts in this case were—facts about Mr. Cowart's condition, his prognosis, and his desires. Accordingly, we have considered as sources of conflict only the very different values that underlie disputes about how he ought best be treated. It is appropriate now to consider whether this is altogether true. In moral disputations it is more frequently the case than is sometimes appreciated, even by—perhaps especially by—ethicists, that what is at issue are facts and understanding of the facts, rather than conflicting values.

In Cowart's case there would seem to be little disagreement about how badly he is injured or how greatly he suffers. There is some disagreement about his future, but this has less to do with what will be possible for him than it does with whether those possibilities are worth his enduring further treatment to obtain. Here the major dispute seems to be between Cowart, whose assessment of the value of his own future to him one might think most properly belongs to him, and his caregivers, who are understandably more optimistic and inclined to think it worth seeking. The real disagreement about "facts" in this case is one that has been obscured to this point for the sake of considering what values lie behind different approaches to treatment; it is a disagreement about exactly what it is Dax Cowart wants, about what he really means when he says he does not wish to go on with treatment, or even with life. Are his professions as clear as so far supposed? Is he entirely free of ambivalence in insisting on a preference for death rather than more of the life he has known for a year and the life that looms ahead for him? Could it be the case that he is making demands, albeit sincerely, for a great deal more than he really wants, in order to escape from an intolerable situation of powerlessness?

Such questions are real and pressing, and unless we can achieve some satisfaction on the issue of what Dax Cowart really wants, we will not have done justice to the complexity of his situation or the depth of disagreement about how it ought to be handled. Of course it is possible that we shall find here disagreements as seemingly intractable as those that emerged over what values should guide our evaluation of his situation, but that cannot be supposed so until we have at least attempted to get at the facts of the matter.

Dr. Baxter, for one, does not believe that Dax Cowart should be taken at his word. Baxter seems to suppose that Dax does not really want to die, but rather issues such demands as this to his caregivers to make them uncomfortable, knowing they cannot and will not accede to the demands, but thereby acquiring a measure of power over them. It is perhaps in order to exercise some measure of control over his devastated life that Cowart resorts to such "manipulative" behavior. In any case, because his pleas not to be treated and his demands to die may be of this sort, rather than unambiguous and sincere, they may be justifiably disregarded. After Dax adamantly insisted upon being represented by an attorney, that his demands might acquire legal force, Baxter was inclined to take him more seriously.

Dr. White, for another, has doubts about Dax's motives. White sees Dax as clearly competent and does not regard his desire to die as a sign of "mental illness." Nonetheless, he is troubled that a man whose life is salvageable and who could go on to live a "normal, worthwhile life" should be "asking other people to participate in his suicide."[6] White regarded it as part of his job to help Dax see that some part of his anger over how he was being treated and his subsequent demands to suspend treatment were "replays of angry little boy outbursts," continuing rebellion against authority, especially as personified by Dax's mother. And indeed there was conflict between Dax and his mother. She, for instance, was very religious, and wanted greatly that Dax would "get right with Jesus." This did not interest Dax very much. And later, after his release from the hospital, when they lived together, her principles forbade her to permit beer in her house, thus forcing Dax into the childlike act of hiding beer under his bed.

Further, Robert White believed he should help Dax see that better pain control was possible through techniques that Dax himself could learn and administer. Finally, White seemed to think that his obligations extended so far as to encourage Dax to go on with treatment to the point where he could choose to end his life without depending upon others to cooperate in doing so. Whatever his doubts about Dax's motives and conflicting desires, White clearly did not see it as part of his job to "save" Dax Cowart's life.

Does Donald/Dax Cowart
Know Who He Is?

Yet another observer with doubts about the genuineness of Dax's desire for death is Robert Burt, Professor of Law at Yale Law School. In the most elaborate analysis to date, Burt argues that whatever desire Cowart may have for death is less his than it is the message communicated to him by others. Burt has a general psychological theory according to which for each of us our consciousness of self is in large measure formed by our perception of how others see us. Moreover, persons in Dax Cowart's condition—those who are very different, somehow ominous reminders to us of the fragility and tenuousness of life—are very threatening to us. Accordingly, without willing it or being consciously hostile, all who interact with Dax Cowart will convey to him, however subtly, their own horror and revulsion. This cannot but confuse Cowart as to whether others really do want him to live, and if they do not, as to whether he wishes to go on living. The fundamental mistake is in supposing anyone is a wholly separate and distinct self, independent of others and capable of a fully autonomous choice.[7]

As an instance of Cowart's confusion of self and his inability to distinguish desires as wholly his own, Burt cites part of the conversation Cowart has with Robert White on the videotape, "Please Let Me Die."

> WHITE: Now it's, I think, beyond much question that if you were to leave the hospital and simply go home that within a short time you would die from the infections that would spring up from open burn areas that still remain. Is that what you intend and want, to go home and die?
> COWART: Actually, I just want a brief visit to home and I don't intend to die from the infection. I'd use some other means.
> WHITE: That is, you would intend to do away with your life.
> COWART: Yes.

Of course, Dax Cowart was so completely disabled at the time of this conversation that there was no active means by which he could end his life. Here, too, he was totally dependent upon others if he was to die by any means other than passively awaiting invasive infection through his open sores. White suggested that Dax endure more treatment until he could end his life on his own if he so desired, and this helped evoke the deep despair Cowart felt about his condition:

> It's a really sinking feeling. I have always been real independent and I liked to do things for myself. I've had my own ways of doing things and pretty much done as I wished—up to this point. And now I have to rely on someone else to feed me, all my private functions I need help with. . . .

Burt does not conclude that such conversation shows Dax Cowart does not want to die or that it reveals some morally wrong response to his condition. But Burt does believe that such statements, especially Dax's rejection of death by infection in favor of an active means he is incapable of taking,

> reveal both his desire to break loose from the helpless passivity imposed by his accident and his belief that he is inextricably dependent on others, in part shown by his rejection of the only means of death available to him without the active administration of others. His conversation with Dr. White suggests that Mr. Cowart is confused, not so much about whether he wants to die, but about whether others want him to die. At the same time, he appears unwilling to admit this confusion even to himself. (pp. 6-7)

This very quick gloss does not do justice to the details of Burt's analysis, but it should suffice to show why Burt is skeptical about what Dax himself and others might too readily take to be Dax's autonomous choices. The most interesting parts of Burt's analysis are the implications he draws for how treatment decisions should be arrived at in cases like Cowart's. He does not opt for the easy, conventional view that if the patient is confused and somehow less than fully competent to choose, others should—family, physicians, courts, etc. Rather, on Burt's view, such a solution contains a "critical fallacy," for it rests on

> the premise that it is possible for two people conclusively to resolve the question between themselves that one is "confused" and the other is not regarding the capacity of both to define themselves as separate and choice-making individuals. I believe this attempt is ultimately fallacious no matter who the two people may be—whether psychiatrist and patient, judge and litigant, parent and child, or, indeed, a conscious person and a comatose person. . . . [N]o one . . . can conclusively characterize himself as a separate and choice-making individual regarding another person when he is perceiving that person as lacking those very attributes; that is, the very act of judgment inevitably evokes the same confusions in the judge. (pp. 13-14)

Thus for Burt, the proper course of action is to "keep the conversation going." When life or freedom hangs in the balance, no one should assume authority to pronounce decisively what is to be done. Rather, discussion and exploration of the issues, values, conflicts, power struggles, must continue at least until a consensus is reached. Presumably, in Dax Cowart's case this would mean that he continue to be treated in whatever manner is essential to allowing him to continue discourse with his caregivers. And presumably, as well, his physicians, nurses, family, will need to be far more attentive in listening to Dax. The proper function of the law, thus, is never to designate an authorized decision-maker, but rather to "ensure that no one in the transaction—whether a judge, the doctors, or Mr. Cowart—is able clearly to identify himself as the choice maker among them." (pp. 20-21)

Of the three analyses of what Dax Cowart is actually saying and meaning, and why he says and means what he does, those of Dr. White and Professor Burt appear the most insightful. And of these two, the strongest part of each is the doubt it sheds upon our original supposition that Dax Cowart was altogether clear and straightforward in his expressions of preference for death rather than continued treatment and a life greatly impaired compared to what he had known before his tragic accident. The weakest part of each analysis, however, may be in the implicit recommendations of each on how best to respond to Cowart's plight. White would seem to want to urge Dax to continue treatment in much the same mode he has known so far, in order that he might acquire at least sufficient independence and ability to end his life without the help of his caregivers. And Burt would keep the dialogue going, no matter how long and no matter how little consensus is reached, rather than risk a (mis)allocation of power that would further unleash repressed, highly destructive psychological forces. Both responses seem inadequate to what Dax Cowart suffers.

Robert White sees Dax as "rebellious"; Burt sees him as "confused" about who he is and what he, as distinct from others, wants; both see him as wanting death only with some ambivalence. In terms of the analysis earlier developed in this book, there is a slightly different way of viewing some of Cowart's speech and behavior. He is indeed angry, both at the condition fate has put him in and at the kind of treatment he has received, not from fate but from people. This, surely, is an important element in the rebelliousness he exhibits against the treatments imposed upon him. Moreover, the passages Burt cites do indicate something other than anger. Certainly they show despair. But do they constitute evidence for confusion, confusion so deep as to be about Dax Cowart's very sense of self, of who he is, what he wants, what is possible for him, and what the consequences of release from the hospital would be? I don't think so. A simpler view, and one more consistent with the bulk of evidence about Cowart's state of mind and his enduring, consistent convictions, is that contemplation of the reality of the death that would befall him upon release from the hospital leads

Dax Cowart to be circumspect in conversing with White, and probably throws Cowart into a certain amount of psychological denial.

At this point in their relationship, Dax Cowart may have little more reason to trust White than he has had to trust any of the other doctors charged with his care. While he is candid about his intention to die, he may well be vague about how that may occur. And too, he may not want to consider the reality of attaining death by the only means available to him: passively, painfully, and slowly, through escalating putrefacation of his flesh and eventual blood poisoning. Such thoughts must be as fraught with psychological pain as his body is filled with physical pain from his injuries. It is only to be expected that consideration of such consequences would contain a large element of denial. But this is quite other than "confusion" about who he is, what he wants, and what will happen if his desire to be released from the hospital is respected.

But for all this, Burt and White are surely correct in supposing that Dax Cowart's desire for death is ambivalent. Given the pervasiveness of both death denial and the fear of death in the human psyche, how could it be otherwise? No matter how courageous one is, no matter how honest, no matter how desperate one's condition, self-annihilation is not something eagerly to be sought. Human beings are too keenly aware of the temporary duration of life, of life as a requirement for valued experiences, to wish its termination without some degree of regret. And more than most of us ever will be, Dax Cowart is courageous, honest, and desperate. He has compelling reason to want to die, and is willing, even determined, to do so. It does not follow, however, that he should have no regrets, no doubts, no ambivalence in looking straight on at choosing death.

Responding to Catastrophic Injury and a Desire to Die

How then should we—as clinicians, lawyers, philosophers, nurses, social workers, psychologists, relatives, human beings—respond to Dax Cowart when he says to us, "Please let me die"? I have no special wisdom to bring to such questions, but I do have the enormous advantage of hindsight, an advantage not granted to busy clinicians in the midst of crisis. And from a cadre of good clinicians, both nurses and physicians, I have been persuaded that the first question to ask oneself, when confronted with a patient so resistant to treatment as Dax Cowart, is: What is it that this person suffers?

In Dax Cowart's case—as perhaps in most cases—the answer to this question is complex and occurs on several levels. The first thing he suffers, as frequently emphasized, is pain—pain that is for most of us so far from our experience, so intense, so constant, and so durable that we can barely imagine how he functions at all.[8] In addition, however, Cowart is experiencing extensive loss. There is the obvious object of grief, his dead father. But Dax Cowart has lost more than this, for he is now without, and will ever after be without, the body that was so vital to his preferred lifestyle. And this loss foreshadows still another, perhaps the most difficult of all to contemplate and accommodate: the loss of a future that might have been. With such pain and such losses, extending into the indefinite future, it is small wonder that Dax Cowart finds life intolerable. In this category as well we might choose to include the isolation and loneliness so evident in his life. However much others may love and care for Dax Cowart, knowing adequately how to respond and relate to his blindness, to his sensitivity to being touched, to all that he feels and all he has lost, is immensely difficult.

There is still a third kind of suffering impinging on Dax, and that is the newly imposed powerlessness and dependency. Much of Cowart's anger seems directed at this sort of suffering, and well it might be, for this is a suffering that is only partially derived from the conflagration that nearly consumed him. There is much that Dax cannot do because of his physical impairments; but there is much as well that he cannot do because of social and political barriers that have much more to do with the interests, convenience, and choices of others. He cannot, for instance, schedule or even voice a preference for scheduling his daily Hubbard tanking, because the hospital operates on certain routines for reasons other than giving patients a say in their treatment. No one asks him if he wants the radio on, or, if so, what he might like to hear. And worst of all, it appears, no one speaks to him as if he were to be taken seriously—as if his perceptions and preferences mattered. (At least this last was true until Robert White came onto the scene.)

If now we suppose ourselves to have a more adequate understanding of what Dax Cowart is suffering, the next question to ask is: How do I respond properly to this suffering? Here the answer will vary considerably according to who is asking the question and what their relationship to Cowart is. For the sake of this discussion, which occurs in the context of considering the limits to which patient autonomy should be respected and deferred to in medical situations, I will try to respond from the perspective of those who bear primary responsibility for Mr. Cowart's care, namely, nurses and physicians.

One way to approach Dax Cowart's situation is to sort it out as above and address each distinct kind of suffering according to the type that it is. Thus, the pain chiefly requires a narrowly "medical" response, while his losses are "social" and his impotence is in large part "political." Pain control is mostly a matter for those clinicians with the appropriate expertise, who know what medications and techniques are available, who can tread the difficult line between effectively controlling pain and saddling a patient with a burdensome narcotics addiction.

Dax Cowart's losses, isolation, and powerlessness are neither natural nor altogether derived from his injuries. Much of his suffering, and much the more difficult part, is social, imposed upon him by the rigidities of institutional structures and routines and by the insensitivity of individuals. Dax's request for death must be seen at least in part as a response to being treated as an object—as a case, a body to be repaired, a surgical patient—rather than as a complex human being whose own perceptions, values, and desires are to be respected and taken seriously. These sorts of suffering accrue to Dax Cowart because of individual failings, and hence are social, and the maldistribution of power between persons and institutions, and hence are political. The appropriate remedies are, therefore, increased sensitivity on the part of all who deal with Dax Cowart, and reform of the practices and institutions that govern the relations between caregivers and patients.

The problem with such a neat division, of his suffering and the labeling of it into categories, is that it invites as equally a neat division of responsibility for addressing. Thus it might be supposed that the control of pain, as a medical matter, is properly the responsibility of physicians, while the social problem of dealing with Dax's losses and isolation belongs to nurses, social workers, family, and friends. Then, of course, we could consign to hospital administrators the responsibility for structuring the delivery of health care in such a fashion as to reduce imposed powerlessness on patients.

But this will not do, not least because, like the identification of "stages of dying," it invites stereotyping and caricatured responses. Even the most plausible of these consignments of responsibility—pain control to physicians—is unsatisfactory insofar as the experience of pain is highly subjective and a function of many more factors than physical condition. Moreover, even as a pure "medical" matter, pain control is one of those areas in which cooperatively and collaboratively involving patients is crucially important. But the greatest drawback of such a division of responsibility for responding to Dax's various needs by different parties is that it once again reduces him to an object, partially dealt with by different specializations and never regarded as a whole person. He continues to be a "case," as the jargon of the day has it, to be "managed."

The fact of the matter is that it is the responsibility of *everyone* who has anything to do with Dax Cowart to listen to him carefully, treat him with sensitivity, and do what is appropriate and possible to empower him. It cannot be the case that physicians concern themselves only with his pain (and cure), nurses with his losses and isolation, and administrators with his powerlessness. This will be hardly any improvement at all over what he endured throughout. It may not be anyone's obligation to love Dax Cowart or always be patient, understanding, or sympathetic with him. But surely it is the obligation of everyone who has any responsibility for his care to treat him with dignity and respect. Yet this is what sometimes seems most missing during that long period of intense struggle to salvage his life and restore him to a measure of normal functioning.

Let Him Die?

The final question to consider is this: Does treating Dax Cowart with dignity and respect entail acceding to his professed desire to die? And the decisive answer is, maybe! What is clear is that there is no adequate moral justification for lying to and manipulating a person for the greater good of saving his or her life. Or to put this point otherwise: attaining the great good of saving Dax Cowart's life and restoring him to a level of functioning acceptable to his physicians does not justify lying to him and manipulating him, ignoring his competent expressions of desire, overriding his choices, and coercing him to do what others think is best for him. But for all this, it does not follow that nurses and physicians ought straightaway to cooperate with Dax Cowart to end his life.

There remains the nagging issue of how decisive Cowart's wish to die is, and the roots of it. Insofar as there is even the least ambivalence on his part, there is ample warrant for others to seek to persuade him to go on with life. And insofar as his desire to die is connected not to his injuries but to the conditions of his treatment, there is compelling reason to seek to change these in such a manner that he will choose to go on living. Both are appropriate and achievable responses by health professionals; both can be done while showing due regard for the interests and rights of Dax Cowart. Indeed, not to listen carefully enough to Cowart to understand his motivation, and not to change what can be changed that unnecessarily oppresses him, would be neither to show him respect nor to be true to the highest ideals of medicine and nursing.

It is a matter of faith that treating persons seriously, listening to them respectfully, involving them in important treatment decisions, and generally doing what is possible to empower the weak and debilitated, will enhance their will to live whatever other burdens afflict them. But this is faith, not fact. And even done superlatively well, might fail. When it does fail, no one—not physician or nurse, not philosopher or lover—can justifiably pursue a course of action intended to save another's life against his or her will. The only respectful thing to do now is to help that person die as humanely, peaceably and painlessly as possible. This could have been done in Dax Cowart's case.

More for legal than for moral reasons, Dax Cowart could not have been straightaway killed by those who cared for him. But he need not have been aggressively treated against his will and in violation of his rights for the sake of extending his life. The Hubbard tankings could have been discontinued and he could have been heavily sedated. He would have died from overwhelming infection while still in hospital. It would not have been pleasant, for him or for his caregivers. But it would have been morally preferable to continuing to force unwanted treatment upon him.

In the end, one would like to think that the right thing was done for Dax Cowart, that he was persuaded, through more sensitive care, concerned and careful listening, greater efforts to accommodate his choices on treatment modalities, to go on with life-prolonging treatment. After all, he did continue treatment—bathings, surgeries, rehabilitation—and did survive the bleak period following release from hospital. He has had difficult times since, but also many good ones, with friends, family, travel, school, and his other, new activities. He does allow that he is glad now to be alive—albeit with the caveat that he does not think it right that he was for so long forced to go on living. And for the greater social good, Dax Cowart has become one of the most articulate and thoughtful advocates of patient rights in the land.

But for all the good that has resulted from Dax's ongoing life, it remains unclear that the right thing was done in prolonging his life. If, indeed, his "consent" for further treatments was, like that for much of the earlier treatment, coerced, or even if it was given on the basis of deliberate misinformation, he would not have been treated with the respect for his human dignity to which he is entitled, and the right thing would not have been done. If his rights were violated—by lies about what would get him out of hospital sooner, or by misleading information about what surgery on his hands entailed, or just by brute force—the wrongs this involves would not be wiped out by the good that followed.

Robert Burt is right to want to keep the conversation going, and it must, as he insists, involve all relevant parties. But it simply cannot be kept going indefinitely, for a price—a fearsomely high price—is being paid by Dax Cowart in the form of suffering and violation of his rights. Presumably the latter will be mitigated if the conversation becomes less one-sided and there is real openness on the part of health professionals to participate in a conversation in which they allow that their patient's values require respect, and may even have to prevail. Burt is correct in wanting this conversation to continue—or rather, commence—because in principle collaborative and cooperative decision making is both better medicine and better morality than the alternative of supposing there must be a constant power struggle between winners and losers.

And Dr. White is correct to pursue those actions that will empower Dax Cowart, that will enable him to exercise greater control over his destiny than he can as a captive of medical procedures and institutions. But it is too much to insist that Dax Cowart must endure unwanted treatments solely so he might kill himself and leave his physicians supposing that that was too bad but that they had done all they ought to have done for him. Their first obligation is not to save his life, but to respect his personhood, and in the extraordinary circumstances in which Dax Cowart is met, this may mean helping him to die earlier rather than later, painlessly rather than agonizingly.

Dax Cowart is not a good example of a badly injured, enormously suffering human being displaying diminished autonomy. Indeed, to a remarkable degree, attributable perhaps only to unusual strength of character, Dax Cowart preserved his sense of who he was and wanted to be. Most of us crumble much more quickly and substantially in the face of the kind of assault serious illness, pain, and powerlessness launch against our vulnerable selves. Precisely because of the extremes of his suffering on the one hand and the strength of his self-concept on the other, however, his case is an invaluable one for exploring the limits of how far we ought to go, in medicine, in respecting an even fully autonomous choice to prefer death to continued life.

If any generalizations about the limits of respecting autonomy in medical treatment decisions can be drawn on the basis of Dax Cowart's experience, they must be the sort that gives all power neither to medical paternalists nor to medical libertarians. Faced as we are in this case with a grievously injured but salvageable individual, one whose valuing of his life and future is quite different from his caregivers, a profound dilemma arises. To defer immediately to his demand to die would be an unconscionable abandonment of the values of patient care and treatment essential to all the health professions. But equally, to persist in administering treatment to an unwilling, articulate, competent person would be an act of monumental disrespect, an assault on both body and soul. The middle ground recommended here and by others is for the parties in dispute openly to explore their differences, sensitively and sympathetically to consider what is at issue, and to come to some mutually agreeable compromise wherever possible. The greater responsibility for initiating such conversations belongs to the more powerful, to caregivers rather than patients. When this is done skillfully, the chances are that even a most seriously injured person's desire to go on with life will be strengthened.

But, of course, it might not be, and not because of any moral failing on the part of any of the conversants. Some disagreements about how to value an individual life between the person whose life it is and those who would care for that person are incommensurable. In this case, finally, the person whose life it is must be allowed to act on his or her values. Before this point is reached, all have an obligation to find reasons for going on with life. But having done so and failed, it would be better to respect an informed choice for death than to force unwanted life upon another.

X

CHOOSING DEATH FOR NONCOMPETENT PERSONS

Dax Cowart's situation can be viewed as one that falls between a certain paradigm of suicide and "typical" cases of treatment refusal in medicine. His case is like a paradigm of suicide in which, while not suffering a terminal condition, a self-conscious and competent agent judges that life is nonetheless simply not worth going on with. On the other hand, it is like a case in medicine where the judgment is made—not necessarily by the patient herself—that in the face of a life-destroying condition, continued medical treatment is not worth the outcome. Most instances of choosing whether to not initiate or to discontinue life-sustaining medical treatments are made when initiating or continuing treatment will at best only temporarily delay an imminent death.

We have considered various ways of comprehending and evaluating suicide, and we have considered at length Dax Cowart's case and the issues it raises. It is appropriate, therefore, to turn our attention now to something more like a paradigm of life-sustaining treatment refusal in medicine. And since so much of our attention thus far has been to persons who can plausibly be regarded as competent decision-makers and the principles that best govern their cases, it is further appropriate that our concern now be with those persons who are not competent to make their own choices and the principles that can be brought to bear in such cases.

When considering persons who are no longer able or who have never been able to make their own decisions about medical treatment, and when these decisions are so serious as to mean the difference between continued life of some sort or death, we face a most urgent moral dilemma. Both courts and ethicists have struggled, often at cross purposes, with procedures and criteria for decision-making in such circumstances. In this chapter I will suggest that there are several important divisions to be made within the category of persons unable to make their own treatment decisions and that these divisions must be attended to in devising both procedures and substantive criteria for deciding what ought to be done. In doing this, some critical questions will be raised as to the defensibility of certain other suggested resolutions of these dilemmas and considerable attention will be devoted to that increasingly influential notion, both in ethical theory and in judicial determinations, of respect for personal autonomy or personal privacy. Throughout I shall have little to say about the crucially important issue of who the decision-makers ought to be (family, designated agent, physician, courts) for the noncompetent, but in the end I will draw out of the recommended substantive criteria for decision-making the implications as to who these decision-makers ought to be.[1]

A Typology of Noncompetence

It is essential to consider, when struggling with what treatment decisions ought to be made for those who are unable to make their own, the degree and perhaps history of a person's noncompetence. There are four plausible categories here.

First there is the category of *partial competence* of the sort that belongs to children, to the less severely retarded, and to the elderly suffering some degree of dementia. Here we have persons who are not fully competent, not fully cognizant of their situation and alternatives, not fully possessed of the capacity for decision-making, and yet persons who cannot properly be regarded as wholly voiceless and incapable of participating in making important decisions about their lives. These sorts of partially competent patients have different potentials for future competence, with normal children having the greatest potential, the mildly and moderately mentally retarded having some capacity for development, and those in the early stages of senile dementia facing a future of ever diminishing capacity. But these facts are largely irrelevant to the question of what degree of participation in their own treatment decisions persons presently possessed of partial competence ought to have.

In the second place, there is the *potential competence* of fetuses and infants, and of some of those (e.g., children) who now possess partial competence. These may be regarded as beings who do not now have the capacity for making treatment decisions, but can reasonably be presumed to acquire that ability in the normal course of development. What significance attaches to this potential when crucial choices must be made now, well before its development, is a matter of considerable controversy.

In another order of magnitude there is the *lost competence* of once normal adults, for example, terminally ill patients in a comatose state. These are persons who, although once fully possessed of the capacity for choice and self-determination, now no longer have either that capacity or even the potential for its recovery. They have no potential for recovering competence, but like those in the second category who have only potential but no past experience, they are presently unable to participate in treatment decisions.

Finally, there are those who are not competent, have never been competent, and who never will be competent, those whom we might categorize as the *never competent*. Chiefly these include the severely and profoundly retarded, but also some gravely defective newborns who either lack brain capacity for developing competence or who will certainly die before such development.

Persons in the first category, those with partial competence, have some ability to participate in their own treatment decisions, albeit a frequently unrecognized and insufficiently respected ability. Morally there is no question of our obligation to respect this ability, and, depending upon our relationship to the person, perhaps even to promote its development or retention. Our concern here, however, is with those who have no present capacity for participating in treatment decisions, and so I shall put aside further consideration of the partially competent.[2] My focus thus will be upon life and death medical decisions with respect to the potentially competent, those who have irretrievably lost competence, and those who have never been competent.

The Principle of Autonomy

In liberal societies, the value that has dominated discussions of how treatment decisions of the voiceless ought to be made is respect for personal autonomy. Indeed, for both competent and noncompetent persons autonomy frequently has been suggested as the central concern. Since one of the tasks of this chapter is to explore the proper range of application of the Principle of Autonomy, it will be worthwhile briefly to examine the notion of autonomy.

The sort of autonomy that is relevant in the present context has more to do with ability than with disposition, more to do with satisfying a condition for competence and moral agency than with virtue. Persons are said to have autonomy when they are able to reflect about and reasonably select among a range of choices. The requisite notion of autonomy here does not require anything so rigorous as Kantian rationality, as a well developed capacity to discern Moral Law and make one's Will conform to it (as if anyone could do this!). It is sufficient that the autonomous person be able to make his or her own decisions with the measure of independence that characterizes those who can take a critical view of the many social, political, familial, and other influences that bear upon them and urge strict conformity. Of course such abilities cannot be said to exist unless they are sometimes exercised.

Persons who live long enough and self-consciously enough to develop patterns of such independent critical reflection and choice-making develop a uniqueness of their own, a kind of authenticity. This kind of independence and this measure of uniqueness together constitute the autonomy of persons which, in the often evoked Principle of Autonomy, we are enjoined to respect. How central respect for the autonomy of persons is to respect for persons *simpliciter* is highly controversial. If we refrain from interfering with a person's liberty (independence) and authenticity (uniqueness), is this respect for autonomy or simply respect for persons as such? Even without resolving this question, however, there is widespread moral consensus that such respect and deference to self-determination is fundamental to a moral schema—at least to an individualistic moral schema, which alone gets taken seriously in our culture.[3]

Important as the Principle of Autonomy is and as crucial as it may be to resolving some of our dilemmas about treating the voiceless, I will argue that it is not an adequate basis for resolving the most difficult cases. For three categories of competence earlier explicated—partial, potential, and lost—different tests are appropriate to the resolution of dilemmas about treatment for different histories of noncompetence. What is generally regarded as respect for personal autonomy ought to be differently construed or weighted in each of these tests. And in at least one of the tests, appropriate to treatment decisions for the fourth category, that of the never competent, respect for personal autonomy is simply an irrelevant and dangerous consideration.

Treatment Decision Criteria

Three significantly different questions might be asked by those charged with determining treatment for persons unable to make their own choices. These are:

(a) the *autonomy* criterion: What would this person choose for himself or herself if he or she could choose?

(b) the *best interest* criterion: What is the best interest of this person? and

(c) the *moral duty* criterion: What ought this person to do if in a position to make moral choices?

The first thing to note about these questions is that they are all hypothetical. Since by hypothesis the person himself or herself cannot choose, we must ask what he or she would choose, would reasonably choose, or is obligated to choose in each case if she or he could choose. Each of these questions has been suggested as the right test for choicemaking on behalf of the voiceless. It is my contention that only the first two are legitimate, and each of these in different sorts of cases.[4]

Only with persons who have irretrievably lost competence or with those who are temporarily noncompetent can we use as a test for determining treatment what the person himself or herself would choose if competent. This is because, clearly enough, it is only with these persons that we could even possibly know what their choices would be. Those with only potential competence and those who have never been and never will be competent can give us no indication of their preferences because they have never had a capacity for formulating a preference. If we wish to maintain the supremacy of respecting personal autonomy, in the sense of independent self-determination, we have no alternative but to choose what the person would have chosen for himself or herself in such circumstances.

Brother Fox and Karen Ann Quinlan

The adoption of this test is nicely illustrated by two cases that went to courts of law for resolution, the Eichner and Quinlan cases. The Eichner case concerns brother Joseph Fox, who had been a member of the Society of Mary for sixty-six years when, on October 1, 1979, at age 83, he underwent surgery to repair a hernia. While under anesthesia, he suffered cardiac arrest, with subsequent loss of oxygen to his brain. The resulting brain damage destroyed his capacity for spontaneous respiration and left him dependent upon a respirator and in a permanently vegetative condition.

Brother Fox had, during a discussion of the Quinlan case held in the Chaminade community in 1976, expressed his conviction that he would not want his life sustained by any of this "extraordinary business." Again, a few months before his final hospitalization, Brother Fox had reiterated his desire not to have his life artificially prolonged if his condition were ever hopeless. When Brother Fox was in just such a condition, the director of the Society of Mary, Father Philip Eichner, requested the hospital to disconnect the respirator. The refusal of hospital personnel to do so sent the case to court.[5]

Brother Fox could be regarded as having *expressly conveyed* his treatment desires for just the sort of situation in which he can no longer make choices. It is precisely this motive of preserving and respecting the prerogatives of individual autonomy that underlies the Living Will promoted by Concern for Dying and various legislative enactments.

Courts of law perhaps justifiably prefer evidence of express conveyance of judgment when validating a treatment (or nontreatment) decision that results in death. Thus in the Quinlan case, despite some evidence that Karen Ann Quinlan would not herself choose to be indefinitely sustained by a ventilator in a comatose condition, the superior court of the State of New Jersey rejected this as grounds for removing the ventilator. Judge Muir, of the superior court, explicitly rejected evidence of Karen Quinlan's own desire on the grounds that her expressions were "theoretical," concerned cases where she was not "personally involved" and "are not persuasive to establish a probative weight sufficient to persuade this court that Karen Quinlan would elect her own removal from the respirator."[6]

Privacy and Substituted Judgment

The Supreme Court of the State of New Jersey overruled Judge Muir's determination that a decision to remove Karen Ann Quinlan from the respirator was "a medical decision, not a judicial one...[and] is to be left to the attending physician." Rather, the supreme court held, Karen's "right to privacy" (the judicial variation on respect for autonomy) was, in the absence of her capacity to exercise it, to be entrusted to a guardian. Subsequently, Mr. Quinlan was authorized to decide for his daughter what would be done.

The state supreme court went beyond simply designating who should make treatment decisions for the once but no longer competent Karen Quinlan. In attempting to protect the rights of a now comatose patient, it authorized a *substituted judgment* for the patient's own, a judgment to be rendered by someone who knows how Karen herself would have chosen in these circumstances. And the court directed that treatment decisions made on the basis of substituted judgment be those that the patient herself or himself would have made—not that which the guardian may believe to be most reasonable or in the best interests of the patient, not what the patient ought to choose, but simply what the patient *would* choose.[7]

Implicit in this decision is the adoption of a "looser" criterion than that of expressly conveyed judgment. The New Jersey Supreme Court, unlike the superior court, offered no opinion as to the adequacy of Karen Quinlan's earlier expression of desire. In designating a guardian who would best know and most respect her wishes, it allowed for what we might call *situationally inferrable judgment*. A guardian so situated as Mr. Quinlan could be expected to know the character, convictions, and personality of the now comatose Karen; such a person would know what the religious or moral dogmas, if any, subscribed to by the patient prescribe; such a guardian would be presumed to know what, in the total context of the life and life-style of his charge, she would choose even if she had never given any expression of desire heretofore. A guardian so situated, the court implied, could be trusted to discern and abide by a treatment decision compatible with what the patient herself would choose.[8]

This is "looser" than an expressly conveyed judgment, for it is a "constructed" or imputed judgment. Such are familiar enough in law, and ought certainly to be acceptable in morality. If we are really determined to respect an individual's rights to self-determination, the Supreme Court of New Jersey has offered as plausible a means of doing so as one could hope to find. Difficulties with the tests of expressly conveyed or situationally inferrable judgment arise when the test is used inappropriately, on the wrong constituency. As I read it, this is what happened in the Saikewicz case.

Joseph Saikewicz

Joseph Saikewicz was 67 years old when on April 19, 1976, he was discovered to be suffering from acute myeloblastic monocytic leukemia. AMML was then and for the most part is still now virtually incurable. Life expectancy with untreated AMML is only a matter of months. The treatment of choice is a fairly aggressive course of chemotherapy administered over several weeks. While not curative, such treatment is sometimes successful in producing a remission in the course of the disease that typically endures for between two and thirteen months before the disease once again proceeds to its inevitable fatal conclusion. The success rate for achieving even this temporary life-prolonging remission, however, is only between 30 and 50 percent. And while a matter of continuing medical controversy, there is evidence that patients over 50 endure the treatments less well and obtain a remission less often than those under 50. Moreover, the treatments themselves are very traumatic, producing severe anemia, bleeding, infections, and nausea, and frequently requiring extensive supplementary blood transfusions. Nonetheless, for all this most people with acute myeloblastic monocytic leukemia choose to suffer the severe side effects, discomfort, and possible earlier death from chemotherapy rather than to allow their leukemia to run its natural course.

Deciding on what course of treatment would be desirable for Joseph Saikewicz was complicated by two further factors. First, he was profoundly mentally retarded, with a measurable I.Q. of only 10 and a mental capacity estimated to be roughly equivalent to that of a child less than 3 years old. Saikewicz was unable to communicate verbally, relying upon gestures and grunts to make his desires known to others and responding himself only to gestures and physical contact. He could not respond intelligibly to inquiries of whether he was suffering pain. A psychologist thought him unaware of dangers and disoriented outside his immediate environment.

The second complicating factor at the time he was discovered to suffer acute leukemia was that Joseph Saikewicz was, and had been for fifty-three years, a ward of the state. Indeed, for the past forty-eight years he had been a resident of Belchertown State School in Massachusetts. When, due to court-ordered physical examinations for all residents of this state institution, Joseph Saikewicz was discovered to have leukemia, the institution sought to locate close relatives who might cooperate in making treatment decisions for him. Two sisters were found, but neither chose to involve herself with Joseph's care. These refusals and the reluctance of the superintndent of Belchertown to unilaterally decide treatment, sent the superintendent into probate court to have a guardian *ad litem* appointed who would be authorized to make choices on Joseph's behalf.

Confronting the superintendent, and then the judge of the probate court (later, the judges of the Supreme Judicial Court of Massachusetts), were two distinct issues to decide. The first was the procedural one of who would be authorized to make treatment decisions in Joseph Saikewicz's case; the second, the issue of what substantive criteria would be employed in making the treatment decisions. The first was obviously necessary, since Joseph could not make his own choices, and it was initially resolved when the court appointed a guardian *ad litem*. Still, the court insisted upon its right (and obligation) to oversee the guardian's choice. The second, however, was far more complex, and what the court required here emerged only when it reviewed the decision of the guardian and stipulated the guidelines such guardians must follow in making treatment decisions for persons not capable of making their own.

Substituted Judgment in the Saikewicz Case

On May 5, 1976, the probate judge appointed a guardian *ad litem*, and the next day the guardian *ad litem* filed his report. At a hearing a week later, the court reviewed and affirmed the guardian's recommendations. The guardian *ad litem* found Joseph's disease to be incurable, and although chemotherapy was the medically indicated course of treatment, he felt it would cause Saikewicz significant adverse side effects and discomfort. These factors, added to Joseph's inability to comprehend the treatment, and the additional fear and pain he would suffer from having treatment imposed, outweighed any limited benefit he might derive from treatment. He therefore recommended that "not treating Mr. Saikewicz would be in his best interests."

In further affirming and justifying this choice (argued July 2, 1976, ordered July 9, 1976, opinion issued November 28, 1977), the Supreme Judicial Court of Massachusetts held that persons have a "general right to refuse medical treatment for a terminal illness . . . [in] appropriate circumstances."[9] It held further that such a right extended as well to those not capable of exercising it (a commitment to equally valuing all lives and fairness were said to underlie this). And then, most significantly, the court invoked as the appropriate mechanism for protecting the rights of those persons who never had a capacity for participating in their own treatment decisions a doctrine of "substituted judgment."

This is a notion the Supreme Judicial Court of Massachusetts held "commends itself simply because of its straightforward respect for the integrity and autonomy of the individual" (431). It is derived most generally from "the unwritten constitutional right of privacy found in the penumbra of specific guaranties of the Bill of Rights" (424) and specifically from *In re Quinlan*, 70 N.J. 10, in which it was held that a second party, in choosing or rejecting treatment for a noncompetent patient, must decide on the basis of what that person would choose if she or he could (still) exercise choice. In the case of Joseph Saikewicz, a patient who never could participate in treatment decisions, the court said this:

> We believe that both the guardian *ad litem* in his recommendation and the judge in his decision, should have attempted (as they did) to ascertain the incompetent person's actual interests and preferences. In short, the decision in cases such as this should be that which would be made by the incompetent person, if that person were competent, but taking into account the present and future incompetency of the individual as one of the factors which would necessarily enter into the decision-making process of the competent person. Having recognized the right of a competent person to make for himself the same decisions the court made in this case, the question is, do the facts on the record support the proposition that Saikewicz himself would have made the decision under the standard set forth. We believe they do. (431)

In promulgating this version of substituted judgment as the appropriate criterion by which to make treatment decisions for noncompetent persons, the court was not yet finished. It had more to say about the procedures to follow with respect to who should use this standard. What it said was, "The Probate Court is the proper forum in which to determine the need for the appointment of a guardian or a guardian *ad litem*. It is also the proper tribunal to determine the best interests of a ward." And going still further, implying that not only treatment decisions for noncompetent wards of the state were the court's prerogative, but that such decisions for any noncompetent citizen were the court's function, the Supreme Judicial Court of Massachusetts held finally that:

> We do not view the judicial resolution of this most difficult and awesome question—whether potentially life-prolonging treatment should be withheld from a person incapable of making his own decision—as constituting a "gratuitous encroachment" on the domain of medical expertise. Rather, such questions of life and death seem to us to require the process of detached but passionate investigation and decision that forms the ideal on which the judicial branch of government was created. Achieving this ideal is our responsibility and that of the lower court, and is not to be entrusted to any other group purporting to represent the "morality and conscience of our society," no matter how highly motivated or impressively constituted. (435)

Evaluating the Court's Decision

There is no fault to be found, I think, with the good intentions of the courts to do what was best for Joseph Saikewicz, showing due regard for his interests as well as his rights. A careful, reasonable attempt was made to determine what would be best for Joseph Saikewicz and to act expeditiously in attaining this end. Testimony was solicited and heeded from attending physicians, from Saikewicz's caregivers, even from a consulting psychologist. The courts were adamant in their insistence that Saikewicz's life and rights were in no way to be diminished because of his mental handicap or his age.

Yet for all this, there is much to criticize in the reasoning and attitudes of the court on how best to make treatment decisions for a patient like Joseph Saikewicz who is not and never has been capable of making his own. And in terms of precedent-setting case law, the Saikewicz case is an especially unfortunate one, perhaps one that, already, has proven to be disastrous.

The first, and arguably most serious, mistake of the courts is their application of a "substituted judgment" test for ascertaining Saikewicz's best interests. There are two distinct problems here, one simply a confusion, the other bordering upon incoherency. Throughout, the Supreme Judicial Court of Massachusetts speaks as if what would be best for Joseph Saikewicz is precisely what he would choose for himself (were he capable of choosing for himself). But whatever a person's mental capacity may be, his or her own preferences and choices are not necessarily identical with what would be ultimately beneficial for that person. To be sure, an important part of what often makes something good for one is that one freely, autonomously chooses it. But there are some things that are good for us independently of our choosing them—e.g., painful medical procedures which are necessary to restoring health, or, say, for children, spinach, where neither would be eagerly chosen despite the desired goal of good health. Yet it is precisely because of this all too frequent conflict between what is best for us and what we would choose for ourselves that we must keep them separate. Extreme libertarians will always prefer self-directed choices over best interests; extreme paternalists, best interests over liberty. The rest of us will recognize the difficult choices that need to be made and the variety of considerations to be balanced. All of us would do well to keep the differences in mind. The Supreme Judicial Court of Massachusetts fails to do so when it speaks, as it frequently does, as if what would be best for Joseph Saikewicz is just what he would himself, if able, choose.

But if this failure to observe an obvious distinction is a confusion, the notion of substituted judgment the court works with is more seriously flawed, perhaps to the point of incoherence. Recall that substituted judgment was a notion first invoked in the case of Karen Ann Quinlan, where the Supreme Court of New Jersey held that once a person was no longer capable of making her own decisions concerning life-prolonging but not restorative medical interventions it was entirely appropriate that someone else make these choices on her behalf. Moreover, the court there held that the appropriate decision-maker would be someone who knew Karen Quinlan well, who knew her beliefs, her tastes, her character; who knew specifically what she might herself have chosen before being rendered incapable of choice; and who, most important, would likely make the choice Karen Ann Quinlan herself would have made under the circumstances. This is what I earlier called a situationally inferrable judgment. Again, the Supreme Court of New Jersey predicated this view of substituted judgment on preserving a constitutional right of privacy for persons no longer able to exercise such rights themselves but no less entitled to the protections of such constitutional rights for their impaired condition.

Such a ruling was and continues to be an enormously valuable one for all who have suffered and all who fear suffering the indignities of having their dying dragged out by insensitive caregivers or the sometimes seemingly uncontrollable imperatives of a mindlessly driven technology. The control we lose in the last days of our dying or of continuing an utterly meaningless life can be still exercised, the Supreme Court of New Jersey assured, by someone who loves and knows us and who will act to protect our dignity. This extension of the right to privacy is thus a further important protection to all who fear the loss of control over their debility or dying and who further fear becoming nearly unbearable burdens to those whom they care most about.

As valuable as this version of substituted judgment is, the still further extension of it employed by the Supreme Judicial Court of Massachusetts is either meaningless or pernicious. In the name of protecting the equal rights of the never competent, the court requires not merely a determination of the best interests of Joseph Saikewicz, but a determination based upon its peculiar version of substituted judgment. *Per impossible*, the person charged with making treatment decisions for a never competent patient is supposed to imagine herself that patient, then imagine what that person would choose for himself despite his never having done so nor ever being able to do so, and, as if this were not sufficiently difficult, she should remember as well that the person whom she is imagining herself to be competently choosing for is now, has always been, and will always be, incapable of making choices himself. Where the Supreme Court of New Jersey created a "legal fiction" in having one person exercise the rights of another, the Supreme Judicial Court of Massachusetts creates a legal fantasy and logical absurdity in charging one person with exercising rights attributed to another for whom such "rights" never had any meaning. The person making this sort of substituted judgment must do (and of course cannot do) contradictory things: she must choose what she thinks her ward would choose while remembering that her ward cannot and never could make such choices!

Courts as Decision-Makers

The other sort of serious difficulty in the appeals court opinion on Joseph Saikewicz resides in its insistence that it alone is the appropriate body to direct decision making in the interest of patients incapable of making their own choices. There is a galling self-righteousness in the court's arrogating to itself exclusive moral authority for directing such decisions. It presumes that only a mind trained in law and a person who exercises the authority of interpreting law can be sufficiently sensitive to the interests and rights of noncompetent persons as to choose wisely on their behalf. And it makes these claims despite the obvious fact that of all the parties familar with the specific individual whose life hangs in the balance, the court is almost certainly the most distant from and unfamilar with that person. Indeed, it would be a rare judge who has even met the person!

Like many a bad decision, this one moves in two, precisely opposite, directions. On the one hand, in its insistence that only courts are the appropriate decision-makers where there is a question of terminating life-support systems for the terminally ill noncompetent patient, or even, it implies, the competent or once competent patient with clearly expressed wishes in this direction, the court makes it very difficult to do what is often best for such patients, *viz.*, allow an earlier, rather than later, death. On the other hand, in its version of substituted judgment as applied to noncompetent patients, the court makes it easier to discount the value of such person's lives by inviting decision-makers to project their own desires upon another incapable of choice. We do this last comforted by the easy rationalizations that as authorized decision-makers we are really doing only what the object of our choice would do if capable. But since the person who is the object of our choosing is not capable, in fact all we do here is project our desire onto another, and in this there is abundant room for hidden hostility or self-interest to emerge in choosing an earlier death rather than a later one for someone whose best interests are just the other way around. Thus one thrust of the Saikewicz decision makes it very difficult to choose to discontinue life-support systems for terminally ill patients, and another makes it all too easy to do so when such might not be best for the patient. Two recent court cases, each of which invokes one of these contrasting tendencies of the Saikewicz case, all too graphically illustrate these dual dangers.

Edna Marie Leach

Edna Marie Leach was 70 years old when in 1980 she was diagnosed as having amyotrophic lateral sclerosis. Within two months this once energetic woman was admitted to Akron General Hospital because of complications from her terminal disease of the central nervous system. Within two days of entering the hospital she suffered cardiac arrest and was resuscitated. However, Mrs. Leach failed to regain consciousness and was then placed on a life-support system consisting of a ventilator, a nasogastric tube, and a catheter.

Mrs. Leach was maintained on this life-support system for over four months, all the while comatose and in a chronic vegetative state. Attempts to wean her from the ventilator were unsuccessful. When early in Mrs. Leach's dependency upon life-support Mr. Leach requested that the ventilator be withdrawn, the attending physician refused. Instead, he wrote Mr. Leach a letter in which he asserted that only a court could make such a decision in Ohio. Mr. Leach then petitioned the Summit County Probate Court to be appointed Mrs. Leach's guardian due to her recently acquired incapacity. This was granted, and Mr. Leach and the Leach's two adult children then initiated legal proceedings to obtain a court order for discontinuation of the life-support system.[10]

A guardian *ad litem* was appointed and evidentiary hearings were held. Extensive testimony was taken from friends and relatives of Mrs. Leach as to the numerous times she had vigorously asserted, when still capable of doing so, her desire not to be hooked up to life-support systems if terminally ill. Religious testimony was taken that indicated such a choice violated no articles of Mrs. Leach's faith. And medical testimony confirmed that Mrs. Leach was not dead under prevailing medical standards but that neither was she cognitive nor was it likely that she would ever recover from extensive brain damage to regain consciousness. After a thorough investigation into the facts, the issues, and the law, the Probate Court of Summit County—citing both Quinlan and Saikewicz as appropriate precedents—empowered Mr. Leach to direct disconnecting Mrs. Leach's ventilator. It took nineteen days for the hospital to comply, but finally it was done and Mrs. Leach concluded her dying.

There is no statutory law in Ohio (or most other states) that authorizes a simpler or more direct procedure for recognizing and implementing a competent or once competent person's expressly conveyed desire not to be sustained by life-support systems. And while not binding on other jurisdictions, the decision in the Leach case is now precedent-setting case law in Ohio. The precedent it sets is a highly cumbersome one, and one that extends to other court decisions in which authority has been expropriated for making life-prolonging or death-hastening decisions for terminally ill persons.

While there might be some justification for courts exercising such authority over long-term noncompetent wards of the state, it is clear that when they do so for others the consequences are sometimes disastrous and always very burdensome for patients, families, physicians, and caregivers. Moreover, the mere assertion of such court authority has a profoundly chilling effect upon patient-physician relationships, as witnessed to in the letter written by Mrs. Leach's physician to her husband. It is always difficult to sustain trust, mutual respect, and open communication where life and death hang in the balance. It is thus no service to those who have made their desires clearly known with respect to using life-supporting technology in cases of terminal illness to have to satisfy courts of law as well as their physicians before their will is respected. We are none of us more secure in the protection of our rights and interests for having courts necessarily involved in these matters rather than relying upon the more direct relations between patients, families, and caregivers.

Mary Hier

Burdensome and undesirable as the intervention of courts is in these matters, the other aspect of the Saikewicz decision—its interpretation and application of substituted judgment—is potentially more pernicious. This danger is grimly demonstrated by the case of Mary Hier. In 1964 Mrs. Hier was transferred from a New York psychiatric hospital where she had been for fifty-seven years to a Massachusetts nursing home. New York continued to pay for her care as she had no relatives that could be contacted. Mary Hier believed herself to be the Queen of England and suffered as well senile dementia, a hiatal hernia, and a cervical diverticulum. These last two together meant that she could take food neither orally nor through a nasogastric tube, thus necessitating nourishment through a surgically implanted tube into her stomach.

By 1984 Mrs. Hier, 92 years old, resisted both injections of thorazine for her mental illness and the g-tube for feeding. She objected to needles and on at least three occasions over the previous ten years had pulled out her g-tube. The last time she removed the tube it was not discovered in time to simply reinsert and would thus require further surgery to replace. The nursing home applied to the probate court for appointment of a guardian to authorize psychotropic drugs and surgery for a new feeding tube.

There is no dispute in this case about the appropriateness of a probate court's involvement. What is problematical is the judgment rendered and the criteria used to justify that judgment. The probate judge, unsurprisingly, found Mary Hier incapable of making her own judgments. He then authorized the administration of thorazine, but not surgery to replace the g-tube. The court arrived at this decision by attempting to "don the mental mantle of the incompetent and substitute itself as nearly as possible for the individual in the decision making process." So doing, the judge determined Mrs. Hier would choose to continue thorazine because, despite the objectionable injections, it would calm her and increase communicativeness. But the gastrotomy, he reasoned, she would reject because it is intrusive and burdensome, she clearly did not want it, and some physicians thought it "inappropriate." Presumably the court thought Mrs. Hier would object less to death by starvation. The Massachusetts Appeals Court considered only the issue of the gastrotomy and upheld the probate court.[11]

In commenting on the appeals court decision, George Annas character-izes it in the following way:

> In an almost self-congratulatory tone focusing on autonomy, the court ac-tually uses the "right to refuse treatment" to deny treatment to a patient whom some physicians find troublesome. This sleight of hand is per-formed by declaring that Mrs. Hier is incompetent to make medical deci-sions for herself; nonetheless, her ambiguous, incompetent statements and actions are used as a pretext for ruling against the very thing that Mas-sachusetts hoped to avoid by adopting the substituted-judgment doc-trine: it devalues the life of the mentally retarded, senile, and severely men-tally ill.[12]

The appeals court justifies its denial of life-prolonging treatment to Mary Hier by depicting not a mentally ill, senile, and long-term incompe-tent patient, but rather a competent patient dying in agony:

> Mrs. Hier's repeated dislodgments of gastric tubes, her resistance to at-tempts to insert a nasogastric tube, and her opposition to surgery all may be seen as a plea for privacy and personal dignity by a ninety-two year old person who is seriously ill and for whom life has little left to offer. (209)

The attribution of a right where the possession of it is burdensome, the exercise of it impossible, and the imposition of it very often deadly is asserting a right that any of us would be better off without. Yet this is precisely the case with according to never competent persons a right to de-cline life-prolonging treatments as an instance of their more general right to privacy and where such a right is exercised through the mecha-nism of substituted judgment. As applied to long-term noncompetent per-sons, this doctrine is not simply muddled, but, as its use in Mary Hier's case illustrates, pernicious. The solution, at least in courts of law and in theory, is a simple and straightforward one: abandon this growing prac-tice and return to the older and simpler standard of ascertaining a noncompetent person's best interests. Were this latter standard used in Mary Hier's case, it would be far more difficult to justify a decision not to reimplant her feeding tube (although, surely, given enough good evi-dence, not impossible to do).[13]

Autonomy Versus Best Interests—I

Two different ethical orientations are vying for our loyalty here, as else-where. On the one hand, respect for persons requires respect for per-sonal autonomy, for maximizing self-determination and individual lib-erty. On the other hand, concern and compassion for persons in need, especially the impaired, vulnerable, and suffering among us, compels us to consider what is best for such persons. Frequently enough, what is best for persons is quite other than respecting personal autonomy, the more so where someone's capacity for autonomy is diminished (Mary Hier) or lost (Edna Marie Leach) or never was (Joseph Saikewicz). Some further consideration is therefore needed on when to use a "best interests criterion" rather than an "autonomy criterion" in making choices for noncompetent persons.

The best interest criterion is more complicated and more difficult to apply than the autonomy criterion. The chief reason for this is that in our usual way of thinking of a (competent) person's best interests, the capacity for and the exercise of autonomy are conceptually linked to one's best interests. For each of us, a large part of what makes something good for us is just that we have freely, autonomously chosen it. One of the most serious deprivations of the never competent, and one of the greatest losses suffered by the once competent, is exclusion from the essentially human task of making personal choices that are constitutive of one's own good. Thus the notion of best interests that ought always be operative in making medical treatment decisions for the never competent is of necessity a diminished one. With no capacity for autonomy, and hence no "interest" in having autonomy respected, developed, exercised, and so on, the never competent must have their best interests calculated on some other basis.

As central as the exercise of personal autonomy may be in the ordinary determination of one's best interest, it is not wholly definitive of it. Some of the other commonly recognized elements within the notion of best interests which are still applicable to the never competent include provision of food and shelter; love and compassion; freedom from pain, suffering, and exploitation; competent medical care; and dignity (albeit a dignity that resides elsewhere than in the exercise of autonomous choice).

A second difficulty with using the best interests criterion is that its application, necessarily by second parties, must be in each case a "reasonable" one. But determining what is reasonable or even what is meant by "reasonable" in life or death medical decisions concerning the noncompetent patient is at the core of the problem. Substantively, let us assume, for the sake of the argument, that action in the interest of the patient is what is reasonable, that is, that the patient's best interests have priority over all other interests. But procedurally, how do we determine these interests and what to do? Is the reasonable choice what a hypothetical "prudent" person would choose, or what "most people" would choose? Is it what results from the convoluted test suggested by the Massachusetts Supreme Judicial Court, or is it what is discovered by an inquiry into the (natural) moral obligations of the never competent? This is a difficult question, the resolution of which goes beyond the scope of this chapter. But I mention it here because it is worth remembering how extremely difficult it is to discern (or choose?) the best interests of another who cannot himself or herself participate in such deliberations. And these difficulties go beyond the usual ones of trusting second-party motives in determining another's interests.

In holding that the criterion of reasonably calculating the best interests of a never competent patient is the appropriate criterion in making life and death treatment decisions for such patients, I am acutely aware that the interests of such persons are significantly different from those of competent, potentially competent, and even once competent persons. But this is in no way to suggest that these interests are less deserving of respect than the somewhat more complex interests of others. Precisely what form respect for the interests of never competent persons must take in an infinite variety of different situations is among the most vexing of all problems in medical morality as well as social policy.

Autonomy versus Best Interests—II

As distinctive as the autonomy and best interest criteria are for treatment decisions concerning noncompetent patients, and as generally separable as are their proper spheres of application, it is an interesting question as to when the one may be used in a situation where the other is generally correct. I have criticized decisions (the first Quinlan case, Saikewicz) where the wrong test has been used; but are there ever instances when, for instance, it would be permissible to use the autonomy test on a permanently noncompetent patient, or the best interest test on a patient who when competent had expressly or inferentially indicated his desires for the present situation in which he is now noncompetent? I can think of no possible cases of the former sort. All such cases land us in the tortured reasoning and incoherences of the Massachusetts court considering Joseph Saikewicz. But cases of the latter sort are not difficult to discover or imagine.

Imagine someone so fearful of dying or of what he supposes will be his fate after death that, while alive and fully competent, he insists that if he should ever be irreversibly comatose he desires every possible measure taken to prolong his biological processes. (Such vitalist views are not as rare as we sometimes suppose, and one is not, by any measure, not competent to make his own medical treatment decisions in virtue of holding them.) Or, conversely, imagine someone so generally reckless about his own welfare as to be deeply self-destructive, if not outright suicidal. In crisis situations involving these persons and of the sort under consideration, we can find an expressly conveyed judgment on the part of our first patient to have his biological life sustained, no matter what the financial and emotional costs to survivors, and a situationally inferrable judgment concerning the second patient to have little or no effort made to sustain his life, no matter how restorable it may be. Are we morally bound to respect these sorts of choices?

It is a simple matter to adhere rigidly to the autonomy criterion when its application results in choices which are, by the best interests criterion, reasonable and desirable; when, as it were, these two otherwise distinct procedures for decision making dovetail in their outcomes. Hence with Brother Fox and Karen Quinlan use of the autonomy criterion results in choices that others would likely make for themselves and which reasonable people regard as in the best interests of Fox and Quinlan. But when, as in our later imagined cases, using the autonomy criterion results in "unreasonable" consequences—those not in the best interest of the patient or those terribly burdensome to others—we might suppose that respect for autonomy is not the paramount concern. Some will be tempted to go so far as to suggest that there is really only one proper criterion for making life and death treatment decisions for the noncompetent, and that is the best interests criterion. On this view, whatever is legitimate in the claim that a person's own choices ought to be respected will be subsumed under the rubric of serving that person's best interests, and autonomy will be respected only when it results in no great harm to others or to the patient.

A second set of facts that incline in the direction of a single best interests criterion for treatment decisions concerning noncompetent patients is epistemological: How do we know what is a patient's autonomous choice? This is an especially acute difficulty with what I called situationally inferrable judgment. For in these sorts of cases, decision-makers find themselves operating with hunches, intuitions, vague recollection of past conversations, and inescapable assessments of a patient's character. The last, perhaps, should be emphasized, because for all of us some of the time and some of us much of the time there is a gap between our opinions, professions, convictions, or judgments and what we do. And if we are called upon to make a situationally inferrable judgment for another, say a parent, which do we rely upon: what we think that parent would have thought should be done, or what we think that parent would have done in these circumstances? Before plunging further into such a morass, one might be better off simply relying upon her or his own judgment about what is best for this person in these circumstances.

There are a number of separate and distinct issues here and it would be a mistake, albeit a frequently made one, to see this conflict as simply one between respect for autonomy and paternalism in medicine. For one of the issues is what to do when harm to others is threatened by following the previously expressed desire of a now noncompetent patient (in keeping someone irreversibly comatose alive because he desired it), and this is not a question of paternalism but one of the legitimate limits to respecting autonomy (or perhaps one of what counts as autonomous choice). That is an issue that goes well beyond the scope of this inquiry to consider, and I will not comment upon it beyond observing that the two usual ways of handling such conflicts are either to define "autonomy" in such a way that no choices that harm others are autonomous or to propose morally justified limits to respecting a person's autonomy that turn on when and to what degree autonomous choices harm others.

Paternalism is, however, the issue when it is suggested that an autonomy criterion be abandoned in favor of a best interest criterion when using the autonomy criterion will result in harm to the patient (e.g., suicide). My own view is that some acts of paternalism can be justified, but that no categorical justification or condemnation can be given of paternalism as such. Nonetheless, the burden of proof for overriding the autonomy criterion where it could be used is upon the one who would override. That burden in the case of persons so severely damaged as to have lost all capacity for autonomy in the future will not be so great as with those persons who retain a prospect for future autonomy, but it is not inconsequential. Paternalism, even in the most favorable circumstances, as where, for instance, it is inescapably thrust upon us in the care of the never competent, nonetheless still requires justification. This is all the more so when the paternalism is elective.[14]

The general problems with paternalism are sufficiently well known not to require rehearsal here. But consistent with this inquiry it is pertinent to note again that relying solely upon a best interests criterion when making medical treatment decisions concerning noncompetent patients will mean that we always use a diminished notion of a person's interests. If I am correct in supposing that ordinarily (wherever it is possible) autonomous decision-making is partially constitutive of one's best interests, (just as it is partially constitutive of one's full human dignity), then to rule out of place expressed or inferrable choices in the name of a patient's best interests means that we are operating with a seriously adumbrated notion of a person's interests. And of course it would be better not to do this whenever possible.

The problem of knowing just what is or what counts as autonomous choice is not so easily dismissed. It is no less a problem because its alternative, paternalism, shares it in the form of presuming to know a person's interests independently of that person participating in the determination of those interests. It is a real and persistent problem endemic to medicine, precisely because medicine deals with people during those times when their autonomy is being most severely assaulted by suffering and personal threat. Moreover, it seems peculiar and inappropriate to enjoin, say, a man's adult daughter to respect her now comatose father's autonomy when she directs medical treatment. We generally suppose that where such relationships abide, the decision-maker, guided by love and concern for another with whom there has been a lifelong close relationship, will make decisions on the basis of her best assessment of her father's interests. Introducing the language of respecting autonomy here seems, at best, ill advised, for it is language that belongs to the cold and formal world of law and philosophy, and not the intimacy of a family.

But the dispute here is largely illusory or semantic. Where close, loving, intimate relationships exist, a daughter's choices for her father's treatment, based on her understanding of his interests, just do embody respect for his autonomy. Where there is a well established relationship of mutual trust, part of that relationship may include the person having previously chosen to trust another to make treatment decisions on his behalf and in his best interests when he is not able to do so. Indeed, establishing and maintaining loving, trusting relationships may well be a large part of this person's authenticity, and thereby his autonomy. In making judgments as to her father's best interests a daughter is respecting his autonomy, for the nature of the relationship is such that the father's authenticity is tied up with the trust he invests in his daughter to continue caring for him when he is poorly situated to reciprocate or to care for himself. It is not merely that the best interests and autonomy criteria dovetail here in their results; rather, a daughter's using the best interest criterion is plausibly construed as respecting her father's autonomous choice, his choice to trust her.

Potential Competence

Conspicuously absent in the discussion so far has been consideration of those with potential competence. One explanation for this is simply that mere potential competence, like mere potential humanness or personhood, makes few moral demands upon us. Ordinarily, respect is owed to persons with interests in the present moment. But on the basis of reasonably presuming that these beings who now are not competent will be so in the future, we can make sense of talk about present obligations we have toward them. We do this in the same fashion as we presume ourselves to have obligations generally toward future generations, viz., by assuming that there will be future generations and that it is in their interest that we now preserve the natural environment, conserve perishable resources, seek nuclear disarmament, and the like.

Consideration of those with only potential competence is illustrative of the logic of respect for persons and how the tests of respecting autonomy and calculating reasonable best interests work. Clearly those who have merely potential competence have no present autonomy to be respected. But an important part of their interests—more important in many instances than preventing pain—is to act toward them so as to maximize the development of their capacity for independence and self-determination. A very large part of the reasonable calculation of best interests of the potentially competent is to act so as to nurture the development of a capacity for competency. (This is why even in the case of children, sometimes especially in the case of children, paternalism is problematical and criticizable.) We cannot act so toward the never competent whose greatest interest may simply be the elimination or reduction of suffering. This distinguishes our regard for the potentially competent (and who they will become) from both that of the once competent (whose present interest lies in part in our respect for who they were) and the never competent (whose reasonable interests have nothing to do with independence and self-determination).

Who Decides?

I promised at the outset to draw out of my schema for making treatment decisions concerning noncompetent persons the implications for who the decision-makers ought to be, and in closing I shall do this. My guidelines are rather conventional ones, in that I accept as a preferred mode of decision-making self-determination and as the central commitment of medicine patient benefit; and where these are in conflict, that the first presumptively takes priority over the second. I do this because I believe generalizable moral obligations supercede role-specific obligations. In the context of treatment decisions for noncompetent patients this means that if there is a mechanism available for respecting self-determination, we are obligated to use it. Thus the desirability of expressly conveyed judgment for the once but no longer competent, and even situationally inferrable judgment, lacking the former. Where an entirely substituted judgment must be made, this ought to be done by one who knows best and cares most about the interests of the noncompetent patient, those interests being paramount. In inferred judgments this obviously requires someone with intimate knowledge of the patient, an intimacy born of a long relationship. Ordinarily this would be a family member or group, and the closer and more intimate the relationship the better. But it might well be a friend designated by the once competent patient as authorized to make choices on his or her behalf when he or she is no longer competent. As with Brother Fox, this would likely be another member of the religious order in which he lived his conscious life. Whoever the decision-maker is, however, it is important that the person be possessed of the capacity to detach his or her own interests from that of the patient and make life or death treatment decisions on the basis of calculating the patient's own desires or best interests, as appropriate.

This raises a serious problem with a blanket endorsement of a family member or intimate friend as the authorized decision-maker. The problem is precisely that though such a person might know best and care most about the patient, and be prepared to act toward that person with unreserved goodwill, in virtue of just these characteristics this is a person who will have great difficulty separating off his or her own interests. While empathy with the interests of another is required, too great an identification with those interests is deleterious. This is where it is possible to find an essential role for others in the decision-making process. Friends, physicians, nurses, hospital social workers, clergy, and finally even lawyers and courts can play important collaborative roles here. And where families or designated friends fail in their responsibilities to estimate the patient's best interests reasonably, these other parties may properly intervene as more than consultants.

For some categories of noncompetent patients medical personnel may be in a much better position to make informed decisions than family, for example, as in the case of severely deformed newborns. Physicians and nurses are likely to know best what are the future prospects for levels of pain and suffering and even relatively self-determining existence for such a baby. And parents, suffering both physical trauma and psychic shock, may be ill-situated to weigh all the factors necessary to an informed choice, and disinclined to make any decisions. Medical professionals also often compassionately wish to remove this burden of responsibility and potential guilt from vulnerable parents. These facts may make permissible the passing of that authority from family to physician, that is, it may make morally permissible the parents' choosing to place judgment in a physician's hands. But superior knowledge and even a superior ability to detach one's own interests from those of the defective newborn do not in this case or any other alone warrant the usurpation of decision-making authority from the most immediate and continuously involved parties, the family. Neither does a paternalistic desire to protect parents who have not sought protection justify using professional power to reach decisions. (There are many other ways of supporting parents in these difficult circumstances.) The duty of consultation and caring on the part of medical personnel is great here, but not so great as to warrant wresting decision-making authority out of the hands of the family. Only irresponsible or incompetent choices will warrant this, and only then may courts become involved.

Ideally, decision-making in these contexts is not adversarial and not a power struggle between competing interests. At its best it is characterized by mutuality, cooperation, respect between patient, family, and physician. Advice is offered, questions are asked, discussion occurs; there is give and take, patience and forebearance, shared suffering and time allowed for accommodation to painful realities. But in this world things are not often ideal, and it is important to be clear about who authoritatively exercises judgment about life and death medical treatment decisions in the whole range of making those choices for noncompetent patients. In this context, there is a peculiarly poignant problem concerning never competent patients, because for them most care is institutional care, and of a sort that is far removed from the kind of caring that is presumed to occur within families. We know that in the kinds of bureaucratic institutions that predominate mere maintenance of biological functioning is sometimes difficult, as such institutions generate their own self-interested imperatives and are further subject to the whims and oversight of a frequently hostile or at best indifferent political process. Nowhere are these dangers and abuses better illustrated than in the sad saga of Joseph Saikewicz, whose situation requires of us now one last reflection.

Reprise: Joseph Saikewicz

To return now, finally, to Joseph Saikewicz, we must ask how, if the criticisms and distinctions made here were to be adopted, his treatment would possibly have differed. Would we find it inappropriate for a court to intervene and be the fundamental decision-maker in his case? And would a different conclusion on whether to treat him or not arise from using a best interest criterion rather than substituted judgment?

In an ideal world, we would expect Joseph Saikewicz to be cared for by kind and loving persons, persons who would be with him and know him well, who in the final, most serious crisis of his life could and would choose on the basis of intimate knowledge and abiding compassion what would be best for Joseph Saikewicz. We don't live in that world. The one we do live in provided none of this to Joseph Saikewicz but instead, early in his adolescence, abandoned him to a state institution where he suffered the common fate of the retarded and institutionalized in our society: he was neglected, hidden, scorned, and no doubt abused. Even as late as 1976, it took the intervention of a court to provide minimal medical care to residents of Belchertown.

Thus given this long history of abuse, it is altogether fitting that a decision about life-prolonging treatments be taken out of the hands of Saikewicz's keepers and placed in the courts. It would, in a certain sense, be better if the courts did not have to perform this function, as it is certainly better that they not routinely do so with persons capable of making their own informed decisions or cared for by genuinely concerned and compassionate others. But that was not Joseph's situation, nor is it generally (or even rarely) the situation of those mentally retarded, mentally ill, senile, or severely debilitated among us consigned to live out their days as wards of the state, or, even worse these days, as derelicts on the streets. Courts must act, we trust to protect the interests of the neediest among us.

And if the court considering Joseph Saikewicz's fate had acted with a keen sensitivity and a clear conception of Joseph's best interests, would it have chosen differently for him? This is perhaps the hardest question to answer. There seems compelling reason to suppose, given both Joseph's limited capacity for comprehension and his long history of abuse and continuing neglect, that he would not have tolerated chemotherapy and blood transfusions very well. In a sense, the court was probably right about this, but its explanation or understanding of why Joseph Saikewicz could not tolerate the treatments may have been seriously incomplete. Surely a large part of the fear and suffering he could be expected to experience from treatments intended to induce a remission in his leukemia is accountable for by his profound mental retardation. He simply lacks the capacity to understand why this strangeness and sickness may be necessary to obtain the good of continued life.

But another large part of the explanation for why Joseph Saikewicz may not have tolerated well the treatment for leukemia is that there seems to have existed no one who could help him do so. Given his history of care, ranging from indifference to hostility, who might have sat eight hours a day with Joseph, held his hand, smiled at him, offered some degree of compassionate reassurance? Small children, too, lack comprehension of painful medical interventions but come to be able to endure them, in large measure because a loving adult endures with them. If we are serious in our commitment not to discount the lives of the mentally retarded, we must surely accord them at least the respect and opportunities we extend to children.

Unlike the unchangeable fact of his mental retardation, Joseph Saikewicz's lack of compassionate care is a contingent matter. It can be altered. He may be beyond the point of being able any longer to respond to such care, but this is the least likely speculation of all in a case fraught with speculation. He deserves the opportunity to be treated, as gently as possible and with the requisite emotional support. At the very least, it should be attempted. No *a priori* speculation about how a mentally retarded person will receive treatment should govern such an important decision. My recommendation is that, in the best tradition of empirical, clinical medicine, treatment of Joseph Saikewicz under the best conditions obtainable and with the maximum amount of caring companionship should be tried. If then he does not tolerate it, regards it as torture, is terrified and sick, abandon it. Let him die early, but with less suffering. But first our obligation is to attempt treatment.

A final thought. The tragedy of Joseph Saikewicz is profound and multileveled. On the surface it consisted of living 67 years on this earth with severely limited human capacities—limited understanding, limited experience of joy and beauty, limited ability for human relationships, for sorrow and love and all else most human. And on the surface it lay as well in his leaving this earth the victim of a dreaded and deadly disease. At still another level, Joseph's Saikewicz's tragedy is to have his name associated with a court decision that is confused and ultimately repressive. But deeper than these, the tragedy of Joseph Saikewicz's life was that others did not care for him or cherish him, did not want him about and were not willing to give much of themselves to enrich his days. In the end, the tragedy of Joseph Saikewicz's life may come down to something so simple as there being no one in all this world who could have held his hand, wiped his brow, and offered him some small measure of human warmth while he endured, or tried to endure, his only hope for a bit more of the life that had been, however meagerly, his.

NOTES

Chapter I. Death Mystiques:
Denial, Acceptance, Rebellion

1. Robert D. Stolorow, "Perspectives on Death Anxiety," *Psychiatric Quarterly*, Vol. 47, No. 4 (1973), pp. 1-14.
2. Jean Paul Sartre, *Being and Nothingness* (New York: Citadel Press, 1956), and Martin Heidegger, *Existence and Being* (Chicago: Henry Regnery Co., 1949).
3. Ernest Becker, *The Denial of Death* (New York: Free Press, 1973), and *Escape from Evil* (New York: Free Press, 1975).
4. For a good case study illustrating this claim, see Milena Maselli Levak, "Motherhood by Death Among the Bororo Indians of Brazil," *Omega: The Journal of Death and Dying*, Vol. 10, No. 4 (1979-80), pp. 232-334.
5. Geoffrey Gorer, *Death, Grief and Mourning* (New York: Doubleday and Co., 1965).
6. Elisabeth Kübler-Ross, *On Death and Dying* (New York: Macmillan Publishing Co., 1969).
7. Cf. Avery Weisman, "On the Value of Denying Death," *Pastoral Psychology*, June 1972, pp. 24-32. For a more extensive discussion of the psychology of death denial, see Weisman, *On Dying and Denying: A Psychiatric Study of Terminality* (New York: Behaviorial Publications, 1972).
8. Leo Tolstoy, "The Death of Ivan Ilych," in *The Death of Ivan Ilych and Other Stories* (New York: Signet Classics, 1960).
9. Oscar Cullman, "Immortality of the Soul or Resurrection of the Dead?" in K. Stendahl, ed., *Immortality and Resurrection* (New York: MacMillan, 1958). Also Leander E. Keck, "New Testament Views on Death," in Liston O. Mills, ed., *Perspectives on Death* (Nashville: Abingdon Press, 1969), pp. 33-98.
10. G. W. F. Hegel, *Hegel's Philosophy of Nature*, trans. M. J. Petry (London: George Allen and Unwin, 1970).
11. Elisabeth Kübler-Ross, *Death: The Final Stage of Growth* (Englewood Cliffs, N.J.: Prentice Hall, Inc., 1975). Raymond Moody, *Life After Life* (New York: Bantam, 1976).
12. Clearly when death denial is sophisticated in some such fashion as this it is not readily subject to the objections to denial earlier articulated.
13. Robert Kastenbaum, " 'Healthy Dying': A Paradoxical Quest Continues," *Journal of Social Issues*, Vol. 35, No. 1 (1975), p. 187.
14. Edna St. Vincent Millay, "Dirge Without Music," in *Collected Poems* (New York: Harper and Brothers Publishers, 1956), pp. 240-241.
15. H. Tristam Engelhardt, "The Counsels of Finitude," *The Hastings Center Report*, Vol. 5 (April 1975), pp. 29-36. For a similar view that could be called "religious naturalism," see Merle Longwood, "Ethical Reflections on the Meaning of Death," *Dialog*, Vol. II, No. 3 (Summer 1972), pp. 195-201.
16. Simone de Beauvoir, *A Very Easy Death* (New York: Warner Books, 1973), p. 123.
17. Albert Camus, *The Plague*, trans. Stuart Gilbert (New York: The Modern Library, 1948).

Chapter II. Is Death an Evil?

1. Cf. the essays by Robert S. Morison, Leon R. Kass, and H. Tristam Englehardt in Peter Steinfels and Robert Veatch, eds., *Death Inside Out* (New York: Harper and Row, 1975), Part III, "The 'Naturalness' of Death," pp. 97-128.
2. Epicurus, "Letter to Menoecus," in *Extant Remains*, trans. Cyril Bailey (Oxford: Clarendon Press, 1926), p. 85.
3. Samuel Gorovitz, "Dealing with Dying," in Michael Bayles and Dallas High, eds., *Medical Treatment of the Dying: Moral Issues* (Cambridge, Mass: G. K. Hall and Co., 1978), pp. 29-34.
4. Bernard Williams, "The Makropulos Case: Reflections on the Tedium of Immortality," in *Problems of the Self* (Cambridge: Cambridge University Press, 1973), pp. 82-100, and reprinted in John Donnelly, *Language Metaphysics and Death* (New York: Fordham University Press, 1978), pp. 228-242. Citations in this essay are to the latter edition. This quote is on p. 234. Other discussions of this view can be found in Corliss Lamont, "Mistaken Attitudes Toward Death," *The Journal of Philosophy*, Vol. LXII, No. 2 (21 January 1965), pp. 20-36; Charles Hartshorne, "Outlines of a Philosophy of Nature, Part II," *The Personalist*, Vol. 39, No. 4 (1958), pp. 380-391; and Douglas Walton, "On the Rationality of Fear of Death," *Omega: The Journal of Death and Dying*, Vol. 7, No. 1 (1976), pp. 1-9.
5. Thomas Nagel, "Death," in *Mortal Questions* (New York: Cambridge University Press, 1979), p. 2.
6. Of course some persons do hold that "death is good," but strictly speaking, this is in a context in which they argue this proposition from the point of view of the species. They may then go on to draw normative conclusions to the effect that because this is so individuals ought not to regard death as evil and ought to accept death, views we shall examine in chapter five.
7. Samuel Gorovitz, *Doctors' Dilemmas: Moral Conflict and Medical Care* (New York: Macmillan Publishing Co., 1982), and James Rachels, *The End of Life: Euthanasia and Morality* (Oxford: Oxford University Press, 1986).
8. Phillipa Foot, "Euthanasia," in John Ladd, ed., *Ethical Issues Relating to Life and Death* (New York: Oxford University Press, 1979), pp. 14-25.
9. Gorovitz, *Doctors' Dilemmas*, pp. 153-154.
10. Rachels draws a distinction between "being alive" and "having a life." The former need involve little more than minimal biological functioning; the latter requires a biography.
11. Foot, "Euthanasia," p. 18.
12. Rachels, *The End of Life*, chapter 3.

Chapter III. If Immortality Were Possible, Would It Be Good?

1. A good, brief discussion of these and several other possible theories of aging can be found in Leonard Hayflick's "Aging and the Aged," in Warren Reich, ed., *Encyclopedia of Bioethics* (New York: Free Press, 1978), pp. 48-53. A very readable account of six such theories is found in chapter four of Roy L. Walford's *Man's Life Span* (New York: W. W. Norton, 1983). Thorough, highly specialized discussions can be found in texts on the biology of aging, e.g., G. Jeanette Thorbacke, *Biology of Aging and Development* (New York: Plenum Press, 1975), and Caleb Finch and Leonard Hayflick, eds., *Handbook of the Biology of Aging* (New York: Van Nostrand Reinhold Co, 1977).
2. There is, too, the epistemological problem of how we could ever know we

were truly immortal, as that would require knowledge of a future not experienced or experienceable.

3. Cf. John Hick, *Philosophy of Religion* (Englewood Cliffs, N.J.: Prentice-Hall,
   1973), chapter 8, "Human Destiny: Karma and Reincarnation," pp. 107-117.
4. Cf. John Hick, *Death and Eternal Life* (London: Collins, 1976), chapter 17,
   "The Vedantic Theory of Reincarnation," pp. 311-331.
5. For example, see James Cornman and Keith Lehrer, eds., *Philosophical Problems and Arguments: An Introduction* (New York: Macmillan, 1974), chapter
   4, "The Mind-Body Problem," pp. 237-326. Cf. James Cornman,"A Non-
   reductive Identity Thesis about Mind and Body," in Joel Feinberg, *Reason and
   Responsibility* (Encino, Cal.: Dickenson, 1978), pp. 272-283.
6. The obvious answer to the question "How are we to suppose any of these perceptions to be possible without the bodily sensations that give rise to them?"
   is that such "sensations" are really only states of consciousness, and states
   of consciousness are wholly mental entities, thus not dependent upon minds
   being "affiliated" with bodies. Indeed, one could go still further and suppose that in a disembodied state minds would have access to states of consciousness considerably more satisfying than those available while encum-
   bered by bodies. The *same* sensations might not be available to us, such as
   those produced by pouring a cold beer down a dry throat on a hot summer
   day, but the new states of consciousness available to disembodied souls
   would presumably be so superior that the loss of our old pleasures would
   not be the least upsetting. Or so it might be supposed. But I have claimed, albeit dogmatically, that dualism is false, hence too are such claims as this
   based as they are on assumptions of dualism.
7. Oscar Cullman, "Immortality of the Soul or Resurrection of the Dead?" in K.
   Stendahl, ed., *Immortality and Resurrection* (New York: Macmillan, 1958).
8. Of course this presumes God sees fit to re-create us in an environment that
   is pleasing to us. Many who profess belief in just this kind of re-created, resurrected, bodily afterlife doubt that all of us will find conditions so agreeable. Presumably, some of us will find conditions too hot (or too cold) to be pleasant.
9. Alvin Silverstein, *Conquest of Death* (New York: Macmillan, 1979).
10. Mortality may be a contingent feature of human beings, but it is surely one
    of those "deep contingencies" Wittgenstein worried about. Indeed, the elimi-
    nation of mortality among human beings may well be the elimination of the
    species—not by death, but by transformation so profound we would choose
    to regard those who never die as a different species altogether: *homo eter-
    nus*, rather than *homo sapiens.*
11. Robert Veatch, ed., *Life Span: Values and Life-Extending Technologies* (New York:
    Harper and Row, 1979).

Chapter IV. Fearing Death and
Caring for the Dying

1. Herman Feifel, "Physicians Consider Death," *Proceedings of the 75th Annual Con-
   vention, American Psychological Association,* 1967, pp. 201-202.
2. Sally Gadow, "Caring for the Dying: Advocacy or Paternalism," *Death Education,* Vol. 3 (1980), p. 388.
3. Elisabeth Kübler-Ross, *On Death and Dying* (New York: Macmillan, 1969).
4. Avery Weisman, *On Dying and Denying* (New York: Behavioral Publications,
   1972).
5. Martin Heidegger, *Being and Time*, trans. J. Macquarrie and E. Robinson
   (New York: Harper and Row, 1962), pp. 279-312; Jean Paul Sartre, *Being and
   Nothingness*, trans. H. Barnes (New York: Philosophical Library, 1956), Part I.

6. W. M. Swenson and R. L. Fulton, *Death and Identity* (New York: Wiley, 1965).
7. S. S. Ray and J. Najman, "Death Anxiety and Death Acceptance: A Preliminary Approach," *Omega: The Journal of Death and Dying,* Vol. 5 (1974), pp. 311-315.
8. Aristotle, *Eudemian Ethics,* 1228a-1203a34. See also his *Nichomachean Ethics,* Book III, chapters 6-9.

Chapter V. Is a Natural Death
a Good Death?

1. It is a lamentable fact of contemporary times that the rhetoric of "affirming the value of each individual life" has been coopted by political forces that use it in a campaign to diminish women's rights and choices, viz., the anti-abortion movement. I intend no such meaning by the phrase, but rather appeal to a much older and humanistic tradition in which such notions are central.
2. The literature on "the right to die" is voluminous, the following but a small sample of both scholarly and popular discussions: Norman Cousins, "The Right to Die," *Saturday Review,* 14 June 1975, p. 4; Beverly Nichols, "My Right to Die," *The Spectator,* 8 February 1975, pp. 148-149; Margaret E. Kuhn, "Death and Dying—The Right to Live—The Right to Die," in *ANA Clinical Sessions* (New York: Appleton-Century-Crofts, 1975), pp. 184-189; James F. Csank, "The Right to a Natural Death," *Human Life Review,* Vol. IV, No. 1 (Winter 1978), pp. 4-54; Robert Malone, "Is There a Right to a Natural Death?" *New England Law Review,* 9 (1974), pp. 293-310.
3. Cf. Tom Beauchamp and Seymour Perlin, eds., *Ethical Issues in Death and Dying* (New York: Prentice-Hall, 1978); Karen Lebacqz, "On Natural Death," *Hastings Center Report,* Vol.7, No. 2 (April 1977), p. 14; Michael Garland, "Politics, Legislation and Natural Death," *Hastings Center Report,* Vol. 6, No. 5 (October 1976), pp. 5-6.
4. Dallas High, "Is 'Natural Death' an Illusion?" *Hastings Center Report,* Vol. 8, No. 4 (August 1978), pp. 37-42.
5. Robert Veatch, *Death, Dying and the Biological Revolution: Our Last Quest for Responsibility* (New Haven: Yale University Press, 1976).
6. Daniel Callahan, "On Defining a 'Natural Death,' " *Hastings Center Report,* Vol. 7, No. 3 (June 1977), pp. 32-37.
7. Of course it is possible to subscribe to a variation on this theology according to which one perceives God to be somewhat more permissive about the proper use of sexual organs, such that, for instance, He regards it as "natural" (morally permissible) that they be used also to attain pleasure or express love or achieve intimacy between persons. Such a broader view of God's desires makes it more difficult to regard contraception and many other sexual practices as morally wrong, but it is essentially the same view insofar as what determines the naturalness and moral permissibility of any behavior is whether it accords with God's desires.
8. There is another possible way of looking at the relation between the "natural" and the "supernatural," and that is one we generally call "magic." The magical view of what is natural is the direct antithesis of the scientific view. According to it, the natural must be contrasted to the supernatural, and death belongs only to the realm of the supernatural. Death is not natural, i.e., it does not occur in human affairs except at the behest of and with the intervention of spirits. Magicians (shamans, witch doctors, priests), if they are any good, are adept at fending off these malevolent spirits and keeping death away. On the other hand, accomplished shamans are also capable of calling forth the supernatural demons who bring death. These spirits intervene in the natu-

ral order and cause the death of persons, usually those who have been cursed or who have somehow offended the spirits. A marvelous account of such a world view can be found in Elinor Bowen Smith's *Return to Laughter* (New York: Harper and Row, 1954). These are views that are generally now thought to belong only to "primitive" or "superstitious" peoples. It might be worth recalling that it has only been in the last few centuries of the "Christian West" that death has been regarded as (scientifically) natural; theretofore, its occurrence always required explanation in terms of God's actively intervening in the natural order to impose death upon an individual. Cf. Philippe Aries, *Western Attitudes Toward Death* (Baltimore: Johns Hopkins University Press, 1974); Jacques Choron, *Death and Western Thought* (New York: Macmillan, 1963).

9. Robert Veatch, *Death, Dying and the Biological Revolution*, p. 289.
10. It is ordinarily quite sufficient, in moral argument, to reject a position because it has morally undersirable implications or consequences. Moral judgments are best seen as reasonable or unreasonable, well or ill supported, and the like, rather than true or false, I believe. However, it might be thought that all such judgments rely upon normative or value premises which themselves presuppose that certain metaphysical claims are true. If this is so (I do not know that it is; it might be quite the reverse, i.e., all metaphysical claims ultimately rest on value judgments), then, where possible, the proper philosophical task would be to examine these metaphysical underpinnings of normative claims for truth or falsity.
11. Leon Kass, "Averting One's Eyes, or Facing the Music?—On Dignity and Death," in Steinfels and Veatch, eds., *Death Inside Out*, pp. 109-110.
12. H. Tristam Engelhardt, "Is Aging a Disease?" in *Life Span: Values and Life-Extending Technologies* (New York: Harper and Row, 1979).
13. Kai Neilsen, *Ethics Without Religion* (Buffalo, N.Y.: Prometheus Books, 1973); Soren Kierkegaard, *Fear and Trembling*, trans. Walter Lowrie (Princeton, N.J.: Princeton University Press, 1954). It should be noted that the theological components of this view of nature cannot be an orthodox Christian view, at least not where death is concerned. Christians might well hold that nature is ultimately "good" because created by God, but they will not use this as a premise in an argument to show the acceptability of death, since in Christianity death is most often regarded as an "enemy." Of course it is an enemy that will eventually, God willing, be overcome, but until that day (Judgment Day?), death is to be opposed and resisted.
14. George Orwell, "How the Poor Die," in *The Orwell Reader*, Richard Rovere, ed. (San Diego: Harvest/HBJ, 1956), pp. 90-91.

Chapter VI. Good Dying

1. Daniel Callahan, "On Defining a 'Natural Death,'" *Hastings Center Reports*, Vol. 7, No 3 (June 1977), pp. 32-37.
2. Cf. John S. Stephenson, *Death, Grief, and Mourning: Individual and Social Realities* (New York: Free Press, 1985).
3. Avery Weisman, *On Dying and Denying: A Psychiatric Study of Terminality* (New York: Behavioral Publications, 1972), p. 41.
4. Avery Weisman, "Coping with Untimely Death," *Psychiatry*, Vol. 37, No. 4 (November 1973), p. 370.
5. Avery Weisman, *On Dying and Denying*, pp. 39-40. Cf., "Coping with Untimely Death": ". . . [O]ur task [psychotherapists] is to change calamitous deaths into unexpected deaths, unexpected deaths into premature deaths, and premature deaths into appropriate deaths . . . if we truly accept death as a part of living, then untimely death can be construed as an allotment, not sim-

ply a tragic stroke of fate" (p. 374). Among other things, it might be wondered what is so terrible about seeing "untimely death" as "a tragic stroke of
fate"?

6. The following analysis owes much to J. David Newell and his discussion of dignity in Paul Trappe, ed., *Contemporary Conceptions of Law* (Weisbaden, West
   Germany: Franz Verlag Publishers, 1983), pp. 411-417. For a very different
   view of the coherence of the concept of human dignity and its usefulness in discourse about death with dignity, see Harold Y. Vanderpool, "The Ethics of Terminal Care," *Journal of the American Medical Association*, Vol. 239, No. 9 (27 February 1978), pp. 850-852.

7. Cf. Veatch's discussion of brain death in *Death, Dying and the Biological Revolution*, chapters 2 and 3.

8. Cf. Ronald Dworkin, *Taking Rights Seriously* (London: Duckworth, 1976).

9. Eric J. Cassell, "Dying in a Technological Society," in Steinfels and Veatch,
   eds., *Death Inside Out*, pp. 43-44.

10. David H. Smith and Judith Granbois, "The American Way of Hospice," *Has-
    tings Center Report*, Vol. 12, No. 2 (April 1982), pp. 8-10; Charles Corr
    and Donna Corr, eds., *Hospice Care: Principles and Practices* (New York:
    Springer, 1983).

11. Alasdair MacIntyre, "The Right to Die Garrulously," in Ernan McMullin,
    ed., *Death and Decision* (Boulder, Col.: Westview Press, 1978), pp. 75-84.

Chapter VII. Suicide:
Choosing Self-Inflicted Death

1. Alvarez observes that the word "suicide" does not even appear in English
   until 1635, in Thomas Browne's *Religio Medici*. A. Alvarez, *The Savage God:
   A Study of Suicide* (New York: Random House, 1970), p. 50. Even today, in
   modern German the word for suicide is *selbstmord*, literally, "self-murder."

2. Alvarez, *The Savage God*, chapter 1.

3. "Anne Marleybone" is fictional.

4. Cited by Tom Beauchamp, "Suicide," in Tom Regan, ed., *Matters of Life and
   Death: New Introductory Essays in Moral Philosophy* (New York: Random House,
   1980).

5. Recounted by Edwin Schneidman, *Voices of Death* (New York: Harper and
   Row, 1980), p. 48.

6. Dorothy Grover, David Malament, Brian Skyrms, *Proceedings and Addres-
   ses of the American Philosophical Association*, Vol. 56, No. 1 (September 1982), p.
   100.

7. "John Rarrick" is fictional.

8. Judges 16:26-30, King James Bible.

9. "Marcellus" is fictional; neither Donatists nor Circumcellions nor this sort of action by the latter is. Cf. W. C. Frend, *The Donatist Church* (Oxford: Clarendon Press, 1952).

10. M. Pabst Battin, *Ethical Issues in Suicide* (Englewood Cliffs, N.J.: Prentice-
    Hall, 1982), p. 166.

11. This is a true story; "Harry Parkinson" is a pseudonym.

12. "Betty Blue" is a pseudonym for a real person. The facts of this case are
    largely accurate; the note is not. But consider this (true) note from Nobel
    Prize physicist Percy Bridgman, who, at 80 and suffering terminal cancer,
    shot himself: "It isn't decent for society to make a man do this thing himself.
    Probably this is the last day I will be able to do it myself." Cited by Battin, *Ethi-
    cal Issues in Suicide*, p. 191.

13. Richard Brandt, "The Rationality of Suicide," in Beauchamp and Perlin,

eds., *Ethical Issues in Death and Dying* (Englewood Cliffs, N.J.: Prentice-Hall, 1978).

14. Emile Durkheim, *Suicide: A Study in Sociology*, trans. John A. Spaulding and George Simpson (New York: The Free Press, 1951); Karl A. Menninger, *Man Against Himself* (New York: Harcourt Brace, 1938). Consider Benjamin Franklin's remark, from *Poor Richard's Almanac*, 1749: "Nine men out of ten are suicides."

15. Beauchamp, "Suicide," p. 77.

16. For an argument in this vein as it applies to Socrates' drinking the hemlock, see R. G. Frey, "Did Socrates Commit Suicide?" in M. Pabst Battin and David J. Mayo, eds., *Suicide: The Philosophical Issues* (New York: St. Martin's Press, 1980), pp. 35-38. For a contrary view of what Socrates is about, see my "Socrates on Obedience and Disobedience to the Law," *Philosophy Research Archives*, 1983, pp.21-54.

17. Such a case was described to me by Tom Marsh, Death Investigator for the Butler County, Ohio, Coroner's Office.

18. Peter Y. Windt, "The Concept of Suicide," in Battin and Mayo, eds., *Suicide: The Philosophical Issues*, p. 41. It is Windt's suggestion that the concept of suicide is best understood on criteriological grounds.

19. Ludwig Wittgenstein, *Philosophical Investigations*, trans. G. E. M. Anscombe (New York: Macmillan, 1953), par. 593: "A main cause of philosophical disease—a one-sided diet: one nourishes one's thinking with only one kind of example." Ironically, despite this general warning, Wittgenstein himself seems not to have heeded it where suicide is concerned. Consider this remark in his *Notebooks, 1914-1916*, G. H. von Wright and G. E. M. Anscombe, eds. (Oxford: Basil Blackwell, 1969), p. 91e: "suicide is, so to speak, the elementary sin." Later, however (last page), he says this: "And when one investigates it [suicide], it is like investigating mercury vapour in order to comprehend the nature of vapours. Or is even suicide in itself neither good nor evil?" The difficulties Wittgenstein may have had in thinking about suicide are perhaps understandable in light of his personal struggles and family experience.

20. Philosophical readers, in particular, may not be satisfied with anything less than painstakingly detailed examination of arguments in support of the principles that underlie categorical negative judgments about suicide. Fortunately, there is available now a thorough, scholarly, and very carefully argued work that does just this. I am referring to M. Pabst Battin's *Ethical Issues in Suicide*. See especially chapters 1-3.

21. Cf. Erwin Ringel, "Suicide Prevention and the Value of Human Life," in Battin and Mayo, eds., *Suicide: The Philosophical Issues*, pp. 205-211.

22. Knowing before someone dies whether to die is their choice is also vitally important information to those who stand in any significant relationship to that person, e.g., as friend, therapist or physician. If there is any degree of ambivalence in making such a choice—as there almost always is—this is justificatory ground for intervening to prevent carrying out such a choice.

23. Betty Rollin, *Last Wish* (New York: Simon and Schuster, 1985); Derek Humphrey and Ann Wickett, *Jean's Way* (New York: Quartet Books, 1978); Lael Tucker Wertenbacker, *Death of a Man* (Boston: Beacon Press, 1974).

24. Kurt Vonnegut, Jr., *Welcome to the Monkey House* (New York: Dell, 1968).

Chapter VIII. The Right to Choose Death

1. Eike-Henner Kluge, *The Practice of Death* (New Haven: Yale University Press, 1975), p. 113.

2. Kluge, *The Practice of Death*, p. 119.
3. M. Pabst Battin, "Suicide: A Fundamental Human Right?" in Battin and Mayo, eds., *Suicide: The Philosophical Issues*, pp. 267-285 and Battin, *Ethical Issues in Suicide*, chapter 6, "Suicide and Rights." Battin also supposes, in her article in *Suicide: The Philosophical Issues*, that "an account which restricts one's right to end one's life in cases in which doing so will have bad consequences for others may seem to oblige us to hold, in consistency, that one is obligated to end one's life in cases where the consequences would be good" (p. 270). But this does not follow at all, at least not for any consequentialist theory that distinguishes (positive) obligations to do good from (negative) obligations not to do harm. The latter is frequently supposed to be a strict obligation, while the former, though good, is not so rigorously required of moral agents.
4. Battin, *Ethical Issues in Suicide*, p. 182; the same point is made in "Suicide: A Fundamental Human Right?" p. 270.
5. Battin, "Suicide: A Fundamental Human Right?" pp. 272-273.
6. Battin, "Suicide: A Fundamental Human Right?" p. 278.
7. Battin, "Suicide: A Fundamental Human Right?" pp. 277-8; Battin, *Ethical Issues in Suicide*, p. 188.
8. Battin, *Ethical Issues in Suicide*, pp. 187-188.
9. Raul Hilberg, Stanislaw Staron, and Josef Kermisz, eds., *The Warsaw Diary of Adam Czerniakow: Prelude to Doom* (New York: Stein and Day, 1979).
10. Battin, "Manipulated Suicide," in *Suicide: The Philosophical Issues*, pp. 169-182.
11. Joyce Carol Oates, "The Art of Suicide" in *Suicide: The Philosophical Issues*, p. 162.

Chapter IX. The Limits of Personal Autonomy: The Case of Donald/Dax Cowart

1. Information on the Cowart case comes from several sources. These include discussion of the case by Robert White, H. Tristam Engelhardt, and Michael Platt, in *The Hastings Center Report*, Vol. 47 (June 1975), pp. 9-12; a videotape made by Dr. White at the Texas Medical Center in Galveston, "Please Let Me Die"; the discussion of Cowart's situation by Robert Burt in *Taking Care of Strangers: The Rule of Law in Doctor-Patient Relations* (New York: Free Press, 1979), where a transcript of the videotape is also reprinted as an appendix; a documentary film, "Dax's Case," made in 1984 by *Concern for Dying*, 250 West 57th Street, New York, N.Y., 10107; a talk Cowart gave and personal conversation with him at Miami University, September 6-7, 1984; and personal correspondence with Dax Cowart in 1986.
2. Of these three possible objects of obligation, I shall examine claims about only the first two. The third—"community welfare"—raises no new issues not already considered.
3. Here a theological claim is frequently made, along the lines that our lives do not belong to us but are rather a trust bestowed by God, to whom we are accountable for their disposition. I will not examine this sort of claim, preferring to stick with the distinctively moral claims that might be made about one's obligations.
4. Dr. Baxter is interviewed in the documentary, "Dax's Case."
5. Robert Veatch, "Generalization of Expertise: Scientific Expertise and Value Judgments," *The Hastings Center Report*, Vol. 1 (May 1973), pp. 29-40.
6. "Dax's Case."
7. Burt, *Taking Care of Strangers*.
8. "I am amused at Burt, physicians, and others who simply refuse to accept that the severe pain which I was enduring was the primary motivation for

my attempting to refuse treatment. Such treatment was so painful that any honest individual must admit that if the treatment were undertaken for blatantly evil purposes rather than medical treatment, it would be considered torture of the worst kind. I am also amused at those who refuse to accept that my severe reduction in physical functioning was an important motivating factor in my attempts to refuse treatment. Why are Burt and others compelled to embark on theoretical journeys in their search for answers that are so obvious? The treatment hurt like hell and was more than I could endure. I believe that many, if not most, victims of severe burns will attest to this." Dax Cowart, correspondence, September 1986.

Chapter X. Choosing Death for
Noncompetent Persons

1. I use "noncompetent" rather than the more often used "incompetent" because of the wider implications of the former and the inescapably pejorative connotations of the latter.
2. This is a large category of enormous relevance. Similarly, so is the category of temporarily noncompetent patients, those who will likely regain competence they have perhaps long possessed after the present medical crisis or diminished competence passes. Indeed, temporarily noncompetent patients may be the most frequently encountered in medicine today. The principles guiding treatment for noncompetent patients developed here have implications for treatment decisions concerning these other categories of patients, but space limitations preclude their being drawn out.
3. Several discussions of autonomy in the recent literature explicate this notion far more fully than is done here. Cf. Tom L. Beauchamp and James E. Childress, *Principles of Biomedical Ethics* (New York: Oxford University Press, 1979), chapter 3; Gerald Dworkin, "Autonomy and Behavior Control," *The Hastings Center Report*, Vol. 6 (February 1976), pp. 23-28; Bruce Miller, "Autonomy and the Refusal of Life-Saving Treatment," *The Hastings Center Report*, Vol. 11 (August 1981), pp. 22-28.
4. In what follows, I shall not directly consider question C. My own view is that it is illegitimate, a kind of moral imperialism most promoted by some few, not mainstream natural law theorists eager to press burdensome moral obligations upon persons least able to discharge them. But rejection of this moral test based on the noncompetent person's presumed obligations does not eliminate normative considerations of what ought to be done in such cases. Indeed, such concerns expressed as what the patient ought to want or do (different from what she or he is obligated to want or do) get smuggled back in under the guise of discerning the person's best interests. Cf. Richard McCormick, S.J., *How Brave a New World?* (Garden City, N.Y.: Doubleday and Anchor, Co., 1981), Section II: "Experimentation and the Incompetent."
5. Eichner v. Dillon, 420 N.E.2d 64 (N.Y. Ct. App., 1981).
6. *In the Matter of Karen Quinlan, An Alleged Incompetent*, 137 N.J. Super. 227 (1975), p. 260.
7. *In re* Quinlan, 70 N.J. 10.
8. This endorsement of the New Jersey Supreme Court's decision should not be construed as support also for its further and confused stipulation that a hospital "ethics" committee should confirm the attending physician's prognosis of there being no reasonable possibility that Karen will emerge from her comatose state to a cognitive, sapient condition before treatment termination decisions are allowed.
9. Superintendent of Belchertown State School v. Joseph Saikewicz, 370 N.E.2d 417 (Mass. 1977).

10. Leach v. Akron General Medical Center, 58 Ohio Misc., 426 N.E.2d 809.
11. *In the Matter of Mary Hier*, 18 Mass. App. 200 (June 4, 1984).
12. George Annas, "The Case of Mary Hier: When Substituted Judgment Becomes Sleight of Hand," *The Hastings Center Report*, Vol 14, No. 4 (August 1984), pp. 23-25.
13. For a number of excellent discussions on the moral issues raised in withholding nutrition and hydration for patients like Ms. Hier see Joanne Lynn, ed., *By No Extraordinary Means: The Choice to Forgo Life-Sustaining Food and Water* (Bloomington: Indiana University Press, 1986). Cf. especially the essays in Part I by Alexander M. Capron, in Part II by Joanne Lynn and James Childress, and all in the Case Study of Claire Conroy in Part V.
14. A far more thorough and careful consideration of when paternalistic overrides of patient autonomy are justified can be found in James Childress, *Priorities in Biomedical Ethics* (Philadelphia: The Westminster Press, 1981), pp. 17-33.

NAME INDEX

SUBJECT INDEX

Date Due

DEC 0 8 1990	MAY 08 '06	
APR 1 5 1991		
MAY 1 3 1991		
NOV. 0 6 1991		
NOV. 2 3 1992		
NOV 1 2 1993		
APR 2 9 1994		
DEC 4 1995		
DEC 3 1 1997		
DEC 2 2 '98		